Craving

Craving

WHY WE CAN'T SEEM TO GET ENOUGH

Omar Manejwala, M.D.

HAZELDEN®

Hazelden
Center City, Minnesota 55012
hazelden.org

Library of Congress Cataloging-in-Publication Data
Manejwala, Omar, 1971-
    Craving : why we can't seem to get enough / Omar Manejwala, MD.
       pages cm

    Summary: "A nationally recognized expert on compulsive behaviors explains the phenomenon of craving and gives us tools to achieve freedom from our seemingly insatiable desires by changing our actions to remap our brains. When we find ourselves wanting something strong enough, we'll do just about anything to get it—sometimes at the expense of our bodies, brains, banks accounts, and relationships. So why do we sometimes have the irrepressible feeling that we need something—such as food, cigarettes, alcohol, or sex—that we really just want? And how do we satiate that feeling without indulging it? In *Craving*, Omar Manejwala, MD, translates the neurobiology of this phenomenon into real and accessible terms, explaining why we just can't seem to get enough. He then gives us tools and guidance to find satisfaction without giving in to our cravings. Dr. Manejwala explains how and why our brain drives behavior, how to change the part of our brain that fuels our cravings, the warning signs that craving is evolving into addiction, why craving is the most difficult component of addiction to address, why self-help and spiritual groups that use models like the Twelve Steps are so effective at changing behaviors, receiving encouragement, and remaining accountable."
— Provided by publisher.

    Summary: "Explains the phenomena of craving in real and accessible terms, explaining why we just can't get enough. Gives tools and guidance to find satisfaction without giving in to our cravings. Explains how and why our brain drives behavior, how to change the part of our brain that fuels our cravings, and the warning signs that craving is evolving into addiction."— Provided by publisher.

    Includes bibliographical references.
    ISBN 978-1-61649-262-5 (pbk.) — ISBN 978-1-61649-461-2 (ebook)
    1. Compulsive behavior. 2. Decision making—Psychological aspects I. Title.
    RC533.M347 2013
    616.89'14--dc23

                                                                    2012047186

17 16 15 14 13   1 2 3 4 5 6

Cover design by Theresa Jaeger Gedig
Interior design and typesetting by Terri Kinne

Contents

Acknowledgments

No matter how cliché it may sound, as anyone who has ever written a book can attest, it's impossible to thank everyone who was involved in making it possible. Many of the experts and researchers whose work I've relied upon are acknowledged in the book itself. I'd also like to specifically thank some of the other people whose contributions and support made this book possible:

My editors, Peter Schletty, Sid Farrar, and the fantastic staff at Hazelden Publishing.

Marv Seppala, M.D.; Jim Atkins; Bruce Larson; Stephen Delisi, M.D.; Pam Shultz, M.D.; Joseph Lee, M.D.; Kent Smallwood, Ph.D.; Sarah Nowak, Ph.D.; Cecilia Jayme; Dave Schreck; Rev. Eygló Bjarnadóttir; Fred Holmquist; Damian McElrath; and the extraordinary team of professionals at Hazelden Foundation who inspired and taught me during my tenure as Medical Director, and who tirelessly give of themselves every day so that thousands of alcoholics and addicts can find recovery there.

Dr. Martha Horton and Tim Leadbetter, for their insights on shame, courage, and emotional maturity.

The Duke University Medical Center Psychiatry residency program, my co-residents, faculty, and staff.

Collectively, the tutors at St. John's College, the faculty at the University of Maryland School of Medicine, the faculty at the University of Virginia's Darden School of Business, and the many teachers who inspired me every step of the way and who really understood that "nine-tenths of education is encouragement."

Mary Beth Schell, librarian at University of North Carolina, Chapel Hill, for her help obtaining hundreds of research articles for this project.

My loving parents, Dr. Bachubhai Manejwala and Rahima Manejwala, without whom no endeavor such as this could ever have happened.

My brother Dr. Fazal Manejwala, whose passion for learning and teaching rubbed off on me at a very early age, and stuck. And my brother Zafar, whose kindness and integrity remain ideals I hope to one day attain.

The many thousands of patients who have trusted me enough to share a bit of themselves with me and let me participate in their healing journey.

And most of all, my sweet, beautiful wife and hero, Cecily, whose support has been unwavering and whose love seems to know no limits.

. . .

Introduction

Have you ever promised yourself you would stop doing something, worked hard to avoid doing it, had no intention of doing it . . . and then did it anyway? Whether it's that diet you were following so well, a promise to your spouse that you would stay sober *this* time, or a vow that you would never gamble your paycheck away again, the inevitable always seems to happen: despite your best intentions, you found yourself engaging in the same self-defeating behaviors. The worst part is, in many cases, you never intended to drink that drink, order that dessert, or step into that casino. *It just sort of happened.*

What explains the mysterious urge to do something that has caused so much damage in the past? What makes that simple thought pop into your mind? When you are doing everything in your power to do better, when you are at your most committed, what brings that powerful image of chocolate into your brain, leading your car toward the grocery store just minutes before it closes? What convinces you to give up what you worked so hard to achieve?

Craving: Part Want, Part Need

Whether it's the smell of the great outdoors, a favorite jazz standard, or the smile on your son's face, desire is a universal emotion. It's the cause of much joy and is responsible for countless success stories. We find it nearly impossible (and depressing) to imagine a life without desire. Our healthy and productive desires are the core of what makes life exciting and fun. Yet sometimes these desires become so intense that they start to feel less like wants and more like needs. When these needs go unmet, you may start to get restless or impatient. After a time, you may become increasingly uncomfortable. If the desire is for something helpful to you, something you really do need, or something that will make your life better, then that's a good thing. It's a healthy craving. But for many people, powerful, enduring cravings are anything but healthy, and they can make life downright miserable.

A good working definition of "craving" is a strong desire that, if unfulfilled, produces a powerful physical and mental suffering. Everyone has experienced this suffering at one point or another, but when these feelings endure or recur frequently, they can be the source of much misery. Cravings are at the heart of all addictive and compulsive behaviors. For some people, it can begin as innocently as a trip to a restaurant, with no intention of drinking, but just to get a meal or visit a friend. The next thing they know, they've ruined their sobriety. For others, it's the "apparently irrelevant decision" to take a different way home from work, a route that just happens to take them past the doughnut shop. Several days later they wonder how their progress toward their fitness goals were demolished. In each case, whether it's the intense, overwhelming, fist-pounding-on-the-bar urge to drink or the ever-so-subtle thought that taking a different road home is perfectly safe, your brain tricks you into repeating self-destructive patterns.

As a psychiatrist and addictionologist, I have seen people work tremendously hard to achieve success only to have all that hard work undermined by what seemed to be simple, innocent decisions. As an expert on the link between the brain and behavior, I've also worked with thousands of people who have been able to reduce their cravings and reduce the effect that cravings had on them by following a few simple actions. These successful people developed an understanding of how—and why—they crave. More important, they took specific and simple actions that resulted in a sense of satisfaction and ongoing freedom from their obsessions. If they suffered from addiction, they achieved more than just abstinence—

they experienced a contented recovery and were liberated from the overwhelming urge to engage in self-destructive behaviors. If they didn't suffer from addiction, they experienced relief from cravings that previously had continually undermined their success. And even more important, when they craved again, they were able to act differently. Achieving freedom from cravings and their effects takes work, but with the right actions, you can get these results.

Today, in the age of media and the Internet, your brain is constantly exposed to images and sounds that can function as cues to trigger craving. "Neural marketers" design advertising with an understanding of the brain and how images and sounds affect purchasing decisions. Billions of dollars are poured into the science of advertising and marketing for one reason: they work. And they work because of your brain and the way it craves. Whether it's subtle product placement in a movie or your favorite television show, or an ad you don't even notice on the sidebar of your Internet searches, your brain is constantly accepting input at a feverish pace. And yet most people believe they are immune to the effects of this exposure and the cues that trigger cravings. As a result, people who are trying desperately to change their behavior are caught off guard when something that they believe is harmless subtly drives them toward doing precisely what they are working to avoid.

And yet the solution can't be simply removing cues. I learned that years ago when one of my patients, an IV heroin addict, checked out of treatment after a friend had accidentally spilled talcum powder on a table. His brain was activated by the image of the powder, and the next thing you know he was out of there. Another patient of mine, an alcoholic Vietnam veteran with post-traumatic stress disorder (PTSD), could not drive anywhere without seeing tall trees along the road that reminded him of the jungle. He described the feeling he got when seeing those tall roadside trees as "proof that I would never fully return home." There is obviously no way to identify and remove all the cues that trigger our cravings, though it is helpful to remove the big ones if you can. This is why bartending is usually *not* a good job for a newly sober alcoholic and why working at a bakery is not wise for someone trying to lose a lot of weight. We'll never get rid of all the trees and talcum powder in the world, however. It's our brains that need to change.

Members of Twelve Step addiction recovery programs figured this out a long time ago. In 1939, the founders of Alcoholics Anonymous described a "strange mental twist" and "curious mental phenomenon" that occurred in *sober* alcoholics that tricked them into taking another first drink. A Japanese proverb states, "First the man takes a drink, then the drink takes a drink, then the drink takes the man." But if this cycle happens over and over, with dismal consequences, what makes a person take the first drink again?

Members of Twelve Step programs have learned that changing their behavior affects both the intensity and the frequency of cravings, as well as the likelihood that they will act on their cravings. Many long-sober members of these fellowships note that it has been years, or even decades, since they craved their drug, alcohol, or addictive behavior. Even when they do experience such cravings, they don't act out on their addiction. Why? What makes them and others who have been successful different?

The short answer is that cravings originate in the brain, and behaviors can and do change the brain. Our experiences, actions, and thoughts produce changes in areas of the brain that are responsible for craving, choice, and decision-making. In fact, the emerging discipline of the neurobiology of spirituality demonstrates that key components of spirituality also affect the brain in remarkable ways. We are learning that spirituality changes the brain and is experienced there. His Holiness the Dalai Lama has focused significant recent efforts, in collaboration with neuroscientists, on the specific ways in which "the mind changes brain matter."

People trying to overcome cravings, whether they are related to an addiction or to another compulsive behavior, can benefit from these same changes. To begin, we need to set aside the naïve assumption that our future decisions and choices will not be affected by our current experiences or that we can usually trust what we think. Indeed, changing our thoughts, actions, experiences, and spirituality—and in the process changing our brains—is what will help us to finally feel satisfied and free from the desperation of not being able to get enough.

The Chapters Ahead

Why do cravings matter? In chapter 1, I'll answer that question specifically. Why is so much advertising designed to create cravings? As you'll learn in this book, many of the strategies people use to reduce their cravings backfire and *actually lead to more cravings*. Cravings matter because they have the potential to lead to behaviors that undermine success, contentment, and joy. Cravings can wipe out months or even years of hard work. Cravings can lead people to throw away all the things that really matter to them in exchange for a short-term fix that is often over before it even starts. Cravings matter because they are powerful, unexpected, and seemingly out of our control. But to understand how that is not entirely true, how we really can eliminate our cravings, we need to understand how decisions are actually made.

Chapter 2 focuses on how your brain drives your decisions. Most people have a basic understanding that chemicals in the brain, called neurotransmitters, affect our moods. What you may not know is that, in addiction, the shape, structure, and function of your brain cells actually change in response to your experiences. Addiction is *not* just a chemical imbalance. Addiction is the result of many complex changes in the circuitry of the brain. The neurotransmitters change, the proteins change, the cell structures change, and the centers of activity (networks of cells) change, making our thoughts and feelings change too. Some of these changes are temporary, some are longer lasting, and some appear to be permanent. In chapter 2, you will learn which parts of your brain are involved in craving and decision-making when it comes to compulsive, self-destructive behaviors. We'll discuss the chemistry of the brain and its relationship to craving, as well as the way thoughts, behaviors, and actions are linked to changes in the brain.

If we never acted on them, cravings would simply be unpleasant, extraordinarily uncomfortable experiences. But it's the related self-defeating actions that lead to so much pain, heartbreak, and misery. In chapter 3, we'll review the link between cravings and actions. We'll answer questions such as, "What makes some cravings lead to behavior changes, while others are just nuisance thoughts?" and "How closely are cravings linked to behaviors, and how do the more subtle cravings affect behavior?" To complete the cycle, we'll explore how destructive behaviors themselves actually lead to increased craving.

People use the word "craving" to mean all sorts of things. We may crave attention, success, love—but we also crave sex and chocolate, or for those with chemical addictions, alcohol and drugs. Are all these cravings the same? What properties do the basic cravings for healthy behaviors and cravings for self-destructive behaviors share? How are cravings for chocolate similar to cravings for crack cocaine, and how are they different? Addiction treatment programs have learned long ago that alcoholics generally cannot safely use other intoxicating substances for long without often succumbing to relapse with alcohol, and the same goes for those who were primarily addicted to drugs. They often say "addiction is addiction is addiction." But many programs for drug addiction allow coffee consumption and nicotine use. Are recovery programs themselves addictive? Chapter 4 examines the relationships between various types of cravings and explains some of the key differences between craving chemicals and craving behaviors. The bottom line is that there are key differences; nonetheless, many of the approaches used to manage cravings in addiction are also successful when working to manage other types of cravings.

Many people do not realize that their experiences, thoughts, and actions change their brains. And these changes are not simply increases or decreases in certain brain chemicals. Experiences and behaviors have been linked to increased sizes of brain regions, increases or decreases in key proteins involved in responding to neurotransmitters, and even changes in the structure of brain cells (neurons) themselves. How does this happen? What do we really know about how thinking changes the brain? A study of monks who practiced compassion meditation demonstrated changes that occurred during meditation. No surprises there. But when researchers went back and studied the monks' brain activity between periods of meditation, they found *persistent* changes—alterations in their brains that continued even when they weren't meditating. Behaviors, thoughts, and experiences have *residual* effects on brain function, which are partly due to changes that occur in the brain. Chapter 5 explores the neuroscientific concept of "plasticity"—specifically how the brain changes in response to input. These changes are critical to long-term freedom from cravings.

Members of Twelve Step programs are intimately familiar with the relationship between craving and relapse, and in this book I emphasize that much can be learned from the collective experience of people in these programs. Many recovering addicts in Twelve Step programs have struggled with cravings for much of their lives while using, and yet so many of them report that it has been months, years, or in some cases decades since they've craved their drug. How have these people managed to dramatically reduce or eliminate their cravings? Successful, long-time-sober Twelve Step program participants have discovered a relationship between things that wouldn't seem to be connected. For example, reviewing your own "character defects" reduces the urge to drink. Making amends, social connectedness, an awareness of powerlessness, and a sense of a "higher power," altruism, service to others, and meditation eliminates or severely reduces cravings. Twelve Step members have learned that these elements must be done together to work. Skipping a few results in relapse in many cases; thus, there is something about the interplay between all these actions that produces the changes needed to eliminate cravings. Furthermore, it seems that, at least when it comes to addiction, a sustained, ongoing effort is needed to prevent a return to earlier patterns of craving and relapse. Why is that? We'll explore the answers to these questions and provide a framework for understanding the basic brain science of Twelve Step recovery in chapter 6. Addiction is a brain disease, and recovery is in part a brain phenomenon, and what we know about just *how* that works is the focus of this chapter.

Whether it's weight-loss support, group exercise, Twelve Step recovery, or even online communities like Twitter and Facebook, people who succeed at changing negative behavior often discover that a group can do what the individual cannot. Even the most strong-willed, determined people can do more when buoyed by the power of a group. Feeling a powerful sense of belonging, identifying with others, and experiencing hope when we see others succeed are just some of the reasons why groups help. In many cases, a healthy sense of competition spurs us to greater success; in others, the self-worth that comes from helping others in the group who are still struggling makes the difference. Each of these social experiences changes us in profound ways, and in most cases, we aren't aware that we are changing. Sure, some of us may feel better in groups (and many people don't), but what we don't realize is how, days or even weeks after attending a group meeting, we behave differently, think differently, and make decisions differently, simply because we connected with others. Each of the various ways that we form connections with other people has a correlation in the brain. In the early 1990s, a special type of nerve cell was discovered in nonhuman primates called the "mirror neuron." These nerve cells, located in parts of the brain involved with planning actions, seem to be responsible for the way that we imitate behaviors we observe in others. In a classic research paper, the Italian neuroscientist Giacomo Rizzolatti and colleagues discovered that some neurons become active whether a monkey performs an action itself or sees someone else perform that same action. More recent human research suggests that these regions of the brain link actions with the observation (or even the sound!) of actions in others. In other words, when others act in certain ways, and we observe or hear them, our brains change. In chapter 7, we'll explore the science behind the power of the group and its influence on behavior. We'll begin to understand how groups influence people in a way that individuals simply cannot.

Over the years, I've treated thousands of addicts, many of whom were downright brilliant in every sense of the word: neurosurgeons, physicists, even addiction psychiatrists who just couldn't stop using. Keep in mind, these are people who are bright, clearly motivated, and in some cases, possess more knowledge about addiction than 99.999 percent of the population. In my early career, even though *I* was treating *them*, they knew much more about addiction than I did. Even so, they just couldn't stop using. Whenever I encountered someone like that, I always asked the same question: "What were you thinking?" That's a question that sounds different to different people. Some consider it to be criticizing, while others hear it as curious. But the answer I got, in nearly every case, was the same: "Doc, I was so *stupid.*" Now, I had tested these people; I knew their IQs. Psychologists may disagree on how to measure intelligence, but one thing was absolutely clear: no matter how you measure it, there was no way to describe these incredibly bright addicts as "stupid."

In other words, the best explanation these brilliant addicts could offer to explain their addictive behavior was *the one explanation that could not possibly be true.* Why is that? How do people who are so intelligent and successful in other areas become convinced that their behavior is caused by something that makes absolutely no sense and cannot be accurate? In chapter 8, we investigate how and why that happens. The correct explanation—that their brains have been hijacked by the disease of addiction and their decision-making with respect to addictive behaviors is not consistently under their control —is so profoundly unacceptable to them that they unconsciously reject it as impossible. In many cases, these men and women had never met a mountain they couldn't climb, and yet they were brought to their knees by a chemical. They cannot accept the notion that they are not in control, and so prefer the explanation that they were "stupid." They believed, at their very core, that they were immune to the effects of the disease. The extraordinarily naïve perception of immunity is at the heart of addictive behaviors—and of craving. It is extremely difficult for people to accept that forces are influencing their decisions without their awareness. And yet, with craving, that is exactly what is happening.

In the mid-1980s, psychologist G. Alan Marlatt, Ph.D., proposed that apparently irrelevant decisions (AIDs, he called them) impact relapse. For example, an addict who finished residential treatment three weeks ago might decide to take a familiar route home from work and, in doing so, bumps into an old friend who suggests they get high together. The addict's brain tricks him into believing that this time things will be different, and so he gives in and gets high. Three days later, when he is lying in a bed on the detox unit of the local hospital, he wonders, "What happened?" As he reviews the events leading up to his relapse, he concludes that he never should have let his friend talk him into getting high. He never concludes that he bumped into his using friend because he walked home the same way he used to go when he was actively using drugs. He never becomes aware that the familiarity of the route was precisely the warning sign. He never realizes that the feeling of comfort was itself the red flag! The apparently irrelevant decision of taking a familiar route home remains outside of his awareness. He trusted his gut. And so, four weeks later, it happened again.

Marlatt used AIDs to describe behaviors that contribute to relapse. But in my experience, there is another, entirely different set of AIDs that contributes to freedom from compulsive behaviors.

We'll explore these *positive* AIDs in chapter 9. Like their destructive counterparts, these positive AIDs also usually operate outside our awareness, but they often make all the difference. Diet gurus learned long ago, for example, that going to the grocery store when hungry is a terrible idea for anyone trying to control their weight. So that's a simple, relevant decision. But several years ago I treated a woman who worked the overnight shift, had breakfast, then shopped for groceries at the discount store near work before driving over an hour to get home. She did this because the grocery stores near her home were too expensive. When she finally changed jobs, she gained weight. She assumed it was the stress of a job change, and that may have been a contributor. But when we analyzed her choices, we discovered that the process of eating breakfast and then shopping afterward was driving her to make healthier shopping choices. She never intended that . . . *it just happened.* We worked together to schedule her shopping trips and arranged for an accountability partner to accompany her to the grocery store. Within a few months she had restored her healthy weight and, much more important, the sanity that comes with freedom from compulsive behavior. Although this is a simple example, there is a set of positive apparently irrelevant decisions associated with all cravings that can lead you toward healthier choices and freedom from craving and compulsivity.

In my experience, that freedom and the sense of satisfaction that comes from making healthy decisions without the pressure and destructiveness of cravings is within reach for nearly everyone. The tenth chapter focuses on hope, joy, and recovery. Most research on cravings is focused on people who are unwell, people in the throes of addiction. What do we know about recovery? What is different about men and women who have managed to gain freedom from their self-destructive behaviors and who are now satisfied and live deeply contented, productive, and fulfilling lives? How do healthy decisions and behaviors sustain and develop these changes? What actions consistently sustain healthy, recovery-based living? We now know many of the answers to these questions, and they form the basis of contented, joyful, and successful living.

At the end of the book you'll find a list of tips for dealing with a variety of cravings. Some tips are good rules of thumb for coping with any craving, while others are very specifically tailored for certain substances or behaviors. It's important to find a strategy that works for you and doesn't leave you feeling discouraged; eventually you'll land on a positive and healthy strategy.

Craving is the core feature of all compulsive, self-destructive, and addictive behaviors. Cravings can undermine years of hard work and dedication. They can lead to heartbreak and despair. In the long run, cravings, and the behaviors that cause and result from them, are truly optional. In the case of cravings, the adage that "suffering is optional" proves to be exceedingly true. Healthy, positive choices and contented living are possible, but require thoughts, behaviors, experiences, and, in a broad sense, spirituality to sustain them. This book explains what we know about how that happens and how you can make it happen for you.

. . .

Craving: Why It Matters

What Are Cravings?

As early as 1899, aromatic spirits of ammonia and hot water were recommended in the *Merck Manual* (a medical textbook) as treatments for alcohol *cravings*. By the late 1940s, craving was described as a symptom of opiate withdrawal, and by the 1950s the term extended to other drugs. For many years since, craving has usually been described as a symptom of withdrawal from alcohol and other drugs. We now know that people who have addiction can experience cravings even after years or decades of abstinence, long after their withdrawal symptoms have vanished.

Everyone has, at some point or another, experienced craving. Craving is a universal phenomenon, and while people may not easily define it, everyone generally knows what it is.

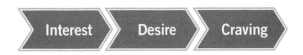

Cravings can be defined as intense desires that produce unpleasant mental and physical symptoms if not satisfied. For some people, that's putting it mildly. Part of the problem in talking about cravings is that people use the word to mean so many different things. I have seen people go to extraordinary lengths to escape the discomfort of cravings, to the point of jeopardizing their health, their family, their jobs, or even their own lives. Like any other physical and psychological phenomenon, cravings can vary in intensity, and they can be brief or feel excruciatingly long. I have had patients describe cravings that lasted weeks, months, or even years. Closer inspection usually reveals that the craving itself didn't last that long, but the experience was so intense and recurrent that it seemed like it lasted an eternity. Most cravings last no more than a few hours, but they certainly sometimes feel like they will last forever.

You don't *crave* everything you *want*. Desire and want are obviously universal, and while people may occasionally (or even often) confuse wants for needs, by and large, the difference is clear. You might *want* a promotion at work, a date with that woman who lives down the street, a beach body, or a better return on your 401(k), but those aren't really needs, and they (usually) aren't cravings. These wants and desires are part of the joys and spice of life, and philosophers and poets have known for centuries that having the material things you think you want may not make you happy. Desire makes life interesting. Friedrich Nietzsche once wrote that "ultimately it's the desire, not the desired, that we love." And the sixteenth-century philosopher Francis Bacon wrote in his essay "Of Empire":

> It is a miserable state of mind, to have few things to
> desire, and many things to fear; and yet that commonly
> is the case of kings.

Wants, desires, passions, and interests are the subjects of philosophers, poets, and religion. They are also the focus of much fascinating science. However, they're not what this book is about. In this book, we will be focusing on cravings rather than simple wants or desires. Cravings, distinct from desires, are truly unpleasant and disturbingly intense, and in this context, are directed toward substances or behaviors that are really not good for us.

Cravings can be much more than simply unpleasant. In addictions (whether chemical addictions like alcoholism or process addictions like gambling), cravings are often the very reason a person acts out on their addiction. Numerous studies have shown that cravings predict relapse or acting out on the craved substance or behavior. For example, studies have shown in alcoholics, gambling addicts, and cocaine addicts (among others) that when people crave, they are more likely to relapse. In other words, craving matters because it actually drives many of the self-destructive behaviors of addiction.

These intense, overwhelming cravings that are core to addictive behaviors are one end of the spectrum, but not all craving is addiction. Rather, cravings come in all sorts of shapes and sizes. There is a difference between an urge for something and a gut-wrenching, devastating, absolute *need* to have it. The simple interest, desire, or even urge to have or do something can of course also be self-destructive. A person on a diet who pulls off the highway on the way home from work to buy a large, sweet coffee drink may not be addicted but is, nevertheless, undermining his own goals and success.

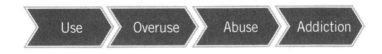

Urges or Cravings?

To understand some of the differences between urges and cravings, it's important to understand the difference between being truly addicted to something (a substance or a behavior) and abusing or overusing it. Let's take the example of alcohol. Some people really want to cut back on their drinking. They haven't lost jobs or relationships because of their alcohol use, they haven't had legal consequences from it, and they've never experienced withdrawal (sweats, tremors, increased blood pressure and pulse). They haven't become tolerant to the effects of alcohol either (needing to use more and more to get the same effect, or experiencing a diminished effect when drinking the same amount that they used to). They just want to drink less.

Perhaps such a person might simply want to cut back for health reasons or because a few glasses of wine in the evenings is interfering with restful sleep. Maybe she doesn't want the calories in that glass of wine, or maybe she just wants to be more alert when interacting with her children. I've actually worked with many parents who were motivated to cut back on their drinking for this very reason. For them, it was important to be more alert and present during the evening hours with their children, and they wanted to be as clear-thinking as possible during those intimate family times.

When a parent in that situation decides to cut back on drinking, say, from three glasses of wine a night to one, several things can happen, and what does happen can paint a picture of what, if any, underlying problems may exist. If you want to know whether a behavior is a problem or not, don't just look at what happens when you do it. *Look at what happens when you don't.* One group of parents in just this situation will cut back to one drink a night and never miss the other two. In fact, they may ask themselves why they didn't cut back before. They'll feel better about themselves, maybe shed a few pounds, feel more alert, and take some pride in following through with what they set out to do. Or they may simply reduce the amount they drink and not spend a minute thinking about it. They never end up missing the other two drinks, except maybe on New Year's Eve or a special occasion when they feel a slight urge and tell themselves, "I think I might like to have another," which they do and then return to drinking a single glass of wine per night, and perhaps not even every night. You probably know many people like this (maybe it's even you): they set their mind to it and follow through without a thought, or even a struggle.

Then there is another type of person who drinks. This guy may decide, for a variety of reasons, to cut back to one drink a day but really notices the absence of those other two drinks. Maybe not at first—maybe a few days, weeks, or months later—but the absence is clearly noted. He may start to tell himself, "I'm not going to drink more than one"; he may make commitments to himself or maybe even to his wife or best friend. He feels the urge to drink more, but he's committed to his goals. He stays at one drink, maybe slips up and has an extra one or even two on occasion, but on the whole he sticks to it. If he's honest with you, he'll admit he often wants another, but his goals are more important to him than that extra drink. He might tell you he craves that second drink, but he can live without it. It's not so intense that he's forced to give in—he can still resist it. It's an urge or maybe a mild craving. But it passes, and he stays on track with the goals he set for himself.

At times in this book we'll discuss the types of mild cravings (properly speaking, these are more "urges" than cravings, as they are milder and rarely yielded to) that this man is experiencing. His discomfort can be managed with some specific strategies to reduce the unpleasantness of these urges and can give him a better shot at a more personally satisfying approach to meeting his goals. But nobody would say he is addicted to alcohol, that he is an alcoholic, or that he *needs* those extra drinks. In these examples, and the others you will read in this book, you can replace drinking with any other behavior you are trying to change, such as eating sugar and carbs, gambling, or Internet compulsions, and the principles will generally be the same. (In chapter 4, we'll discuss how most of these behaviors, when they become compulsive, are essentially the same, and we'll also explore some of the differences that do exist.)

Then there is another type of person who is trying to change her behavior. This person may really recognize she is drinking too much. Her husband may be pestering her to cut down. She may have received a DUI or called in late to work on a Monday morning after a bad drinking bender. Or maybe it hasn't affected work at all, but she did some things she was embarrassed about, such as "drunk dialing." Clearly, she hasn't always been this way. She wonders if it's a phase. The idea of stopping drinking altogether is pretty unattractive to her. She doesn't want to stop drinking forever. She enjoys drinking. She's tried to cut down and she can . . . for a while. Sooner or later, though, she's back to her old ways, and maybe worse. Often, but not always, when she is cutting back on her drinking, or stopping for a while, she experiences a strong desire to drink—a *craving*.

These cravings can take many different forms, as we'll explore later in this book. Sometimes they can show up as an innocent thought: "I can have just one more," or "I've been doing so well, I *deserve* this." Sometimes the thought is not so benign, like "I hate this. . . . I'm giving up on this abstinence idea." At other times, thoughts can be very subtle or deceptive, such as "It's beer, so it doesn't count." At still other times, the craving can be almost *dissociative.* Have you ever had the experience of driving down the freeway and planning to get off at a certain exit, and making a note to yourself to get off at that exit, but then drifting off in your mind and missing that exit completely? Perhaps you had actually driven several miles before you noticed it. That's a close approximation to what happens with what I call "the absent-minded craving." In that case, the person may take a drink without even thinking about it, almost automatically. He has no obvious desire to drink, and no thought of the promise he made to himself, but suddenly he finds himself with half a drink in his hand, because he drank the first half without even realizing it.

It's worth noting that the woman described above may not actually be an alcoholic. This type of craving does occur in non-alcoholics, and some of these cases are described by experts as "alcohol abuse." Drinking leads to consequences, the person still uses, and the cravings can be intense, but some support, some very severe consequences, a strong motivation, or maybe just a change of heart can lead, in some cases, to the person moderating or stopping the drinking. If your behavior falls into this category (whether it's drinking, compulsive eating, or some other behavior you are trying to control), you probably should seek a professional to at least help diagnose the issue and offer some strategies for helping you meet your goals. If this is you, the description of cravings in this book will apply to you, and the explanations and recommendations will be relevant and useful as you make more successful attempts to modify your behavior. You can do some very specific things once you have a better sense of what you are dealing with that can help you change your behavior and meet your goals, and I'll lay those out very clearly so you can be successful.

Of course, these are just examples and many more variations exist, but there is an important one we haven't covered yet—an even more severe type of craving that is generally found only in people who have addiction.

What Is Addiction?

Let's take a look at the word "addiction." Some think of addiction as a dirty word or something pejorative, but it's really nothing more than a description of a set of behaviors that are hardwired into the brain. In fact, it comes from the Latin word "addictionem," which basically means "a devoting." As you'll see in this book, when it comes to addiction, the thoughts, perspectives, behaviors, and even the very neurons or brain cells of the person are *devoted* to the craved substance or behavior. The causes of addiction are complex and multiple, and the types of addiction are myriad as well. But all addictions share some key features, and the most important of those is craving.

People who suffer from addictions experience milder desires and urges as well. Often they drink not because they need to, but simply because they want to. And they also may sometimes experience the mild or even the stronger cravings I've described above. But most people with addiction also experience another type of craving, one that is devastatingly destructive. This is the fist-pounding, can't-live-without-it, absolutely-gotta-have-it severe addictive craving.

This craving cannot be ignored, it cannot be voluntarily suppressed, and it can't be wished away. It often feels like it will last forever and that the only choice is to give in. It feels as powerful as the biological drive to breathe or the thirst for water. It won't allow itself to be ignored until it's satisfied. The tragedy is that giving in or succumbing to the craving and acting out is not the end of it; it often leads, later, to even stronger cravings or cravings for even more. In some cases, giving in to the cravings leads to craving another substance or behavior. It's a vicious cycle that affects more than 10 percent of the U.S. population, and it won't be eliminated by stronger willpower, an ad campaign to "just say no," or any number of scare tactics or legal interventions. What we're discussing is addiction and, sadly, it can be deadly. People with addiction need their substance or behavior to function. In some cases, stopping the drug use or behavior can produce life-threatening consequences, such as seizure or delirium (with alcohol), or the equally deadly refeeding syndrome with anorexia, where suddenly resuming normal eating after starvation can sometimes lead to heart failure and even death.

These individuals cannot consistently use in moderation. Unlike our other examples, where a person could use or act out in a limited, controlled fashion, people with addiction generally cannot consistently control their behavior when it comes to the addictive substance or process. One important caveat is that some people with addiction actually *can* control their behavior . . . for a time. This temporary control wreaks havoc on the mind of someone with addiction, because it convinces him that he has finally regained control. Then later, when the behavior spirals out of control again, it's often far more devastating than it was before. This, by the way, is one reason why experts describe addiction as a progressive disease. Over time, the natural development of addiction is that it gets worse, although there may be periods (often long periods) of improvement.

Yet over the years I've observed that when this happens—when the behavior temporarily appears to be getting better—the mind is actually getting worse, setting the person up for relapse. Here's an example of this *behavior-better-brain-worse* scenario. Consider a guy named "Lance" who struggled with gambling for years. At first it was sports betting, then it was day trading, and these days it's some combination of online and casino gambling. Like most people who are struggling with gambling addiction, he had some winning streaks and some losing streaks. When he won, he knew it was because of his strategy. When he lost, he knew it was temporary—he didn't even really think of himself as losing; rather, he would say, "The casino is holding my money for me right now until I win it back." That sounded bad enough, and it was. However, at one point, with enough pressure and when he was in the hole financially, he finally decided enough was enough. He acknowledged he had a serious problem, even that he was addicted to gambling, and then he simply stopped gambling. His wife was proud of him, his friends (at least the few who knew about his problem) were supportive, and Lance really got the sense that he was free of this issue. He called his gambling "a phase."

From the outside, it would really appear that things were looking up for Lance. The behavior wasn't just reduced—it was gone. Lance was not gambling at all. But let's take a look at what Lance was *thinking.* Lance began to reflect on how he was able to simply stop gambling by putting his mind to it. He looked with scorn on people who needed gambling addiction treatment and at people who described themselves as gambling addicts. He started to ask himself why they didn't just "man up and quit, like I did." He then made a startling conclusion: if he was able to quit on his own when he wanted to, he must not be addicted. Now, mind you, when Lance was gambling (toward the end), he was aware that he was addicted. In some regards, his mind was actually healthier because he knew he had a problem. He had insight. Later, after stopping for a while, he became convinced that he didn't have a problem. His insight was actually worse—his mind was lying to him at a furious pace even though he was not gambling. You can imagine what happened next; because he knew he wasn't addicted, he told himself that he could gamble recreationally, just occasionally and for fun. Before long, he was back in a deeper hole than ever, asking himself how he had let it happen again. Lance's behavior was better but his mind was worse, which is why we emphasize that quitting isn't enough; it has to be followed up with a genuine recovery-oriented program, which I'll describe later in this book. The great thing about focusing on recovery rather than on the problematic/addictive behavior is that not only do your brain and behavior improve, but your happiness and sense of satisfaction dramatically increase as well.

If you fall into any of the above-mentioned categories of addiction, you absolutely should get professional help to assess the problem and support you in developing individualized strategies to obtain relief and freedom. But even if you fall into the severest category of addiction and craving, the explanations and methods in this book will be very helpful as you progress along your journey toward personal recovery.

Cravings Matter

Why do cravings matter? In 2012, craving was finally added to the upcoming fifth edition of the American Psychiatric Association's *Diagnostic and Statistical Manual of Mental Disorders* (DSM-V) criteria for addiction. Doctors are paying more attention to cravings now than ever before. Why is that? There are three main reasons. First, cravings are correlated with relapse. People who crave more are more likely to return to the craved substance or behavior. Second, cravings are distressing and uncomfortable. People who have severe cravings will often describe them as maddeningly uncomfortable. And finally, cravings matter because they can be affected, they can be improved, they can be relieved, and, in many cases, they can even be prevented. Recently, medications and other therapies have been developed to help reduce or eliminate alcohol and other drug cravings.

Some evidence suggests that these medications may also be helpful with "process" cravings, like gambling and compulsive eating. This book will explore the evidence behind all of these options so you can decide a course of action that's right for you.

Perhaps the most important reason that cravings matter is because they are *yours*. They are deeply personal. You can paint a vivid picture of them or even show someone what happens to you when you experience them. But no matter how thoroughly you describe or explain your cravings, you are the only one who is experiencing them. This is very important because, in the effort to get a handle on their cravings, many of the people I work with try to compare their cravings to what others are experiencing. Often, they will either see that their cravings seem worse, and become convinced that they are different and thus cannot get well, or that their cravings are milder, and so conclude, "I don't really need all this help." Either way, comparing your cravings with what other people experience is a losing game and can only serve to undermine your success. As we'll see later (particularly in chapter 7), if you must share and compare your experiences with that of other people, be sure to look for similarities rather than differences.

Your cravings matter because you alone are experiencing them, they are influencing your behavior, and your actions can directly influence them. You are not helpless when it comes to your cravings, nor are you destined to experience them forever. There are specific actions you can take, which I'll describe in detail, that can affect the frequency and intensity of your cravings. Your actions can also reduce the likelihood that, should you experience a craving, you will act on that craving and relapse to the behavior you have been trying to control.

Whether you use the term "craving" to describe a simple urge or desire, or even if you mean the kind of severe craving found in addiction, cravings matter. Whether it's craving for a drink, a drug, a slot machine, a chocolate cake, or a cigarette, cravings matter because they either influence or directly drive your behaviors. But even more important, changes in your actions and behaviors can influence your cravings and improve your ability to get relief and find freedom from the self-destructive things you are craving.

. . .

2

Beyond Neurotransmitters
The *Real* Brain Science of Craving and Decision-Making

Alcoholism: Disease ~~or~~ of Choice

Medical science news is very difficult to interpret. One study shows that drinking a little wine is good for you, while another suggests it's very bad. One study shows that hormone replacement therapy for women is a good idea, while another suggests it can lead to breast cancer. One week the news is eat more of this food, and the next week it's eat less. In the midst of this flood of conflicting information, it's easy to either get an oversimplified (and inaccurate) picture of the science of health and wellness or draw the conclusion that we don't really know anything at all. The reality is that we know quite a bit about the brain and its function, and much of it *is* easily understood; what's missing is basic education about the way the brain works and how its processes affect experiences and decisions.

Most people have heard of neurotransmitters, the chemicals that brain cells use to communicate with each other. Today's news is filled with conflicting information about these chemicals and how we can modify them: exercise increases serotonin, serotonin is responsible for good mood, too much serotonin leads to irritability, too little leads to depression. Television ads for antidepressants might convince you that all you need is a little more of a certain chemical and you'll be okay, as if your brain contained two beakers, one for serotonin and one for norepinephrine, and all you need is to fill up one of the beakers if you are running a little low. Doctors may reinforce this simplistic idea by describing depression as a *chemical imbalance*. "Don't worry, Mr. Jones. You just need some more serotonin because you are running a little low."

In order to understand why you crave and how you make decisions, you need a more sophisticated understanding of the brain and its function. Although estimates vary, most scientists agree that the typical human brain contains about 100 billion nerve cells, or neurons, and at least that many supporting cells, called glia. Your neurons have cell bodies and projections called axons and dendrites. It is often helpful to think of axons as broadcast antennae and dendrites are receiving antennae. The gaps between axons and dendrites are called synapses. When an electrical impulse is activated along an axon, a neurotransmitter is released into that gap. The neurotransmitter then activates the dendrite of the next neuron (often by attaching to a special protein called a receptor) and *voilà*, one neuron just "talked" to another one! (See the illustration below.) Each individual neuron can have many synapses. Thus, your brain is highly networked, and small changes in one area can produce dramatic effects throughout the brain.

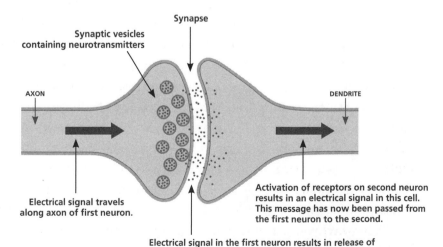

Synapse

Synaptic vesicles containing neurotransmitters

AXON

DENDRITE

Electrical signal travels along axon of first neuron.

Activation of receptors on second neuron results in an electrical signal in this cell. This message has now been passed from the first neuron to the second.

Electrical signal in the first neuron results in release of vesicles containing neurotransmitters. The neurotransmitters then activate receptors on the second neuron.

Your brain has gray matter and white matter. The gray matter of your brain consists mostly of the cell bodies of your neurons and the dendrites. The white matter is white because the long axons (transmitting antennae) are covered with a whitish fat-and-protein insulation called myelin. Myelin helps the electrical signal travel more efficiently along the axon. Your cerebral cortex is the outer part of your brain and is mostly gray matter. Deeper in your brain are nuclei, dense regions of cell bodies. These deeper regions, surrounded by white matter, are also gray matter and are responsible for key functions of your brain. For example, one set of nuclei deep in your brain is called the thalamus. Your thalamus functions as a sort of relay system, as sensory and motor signals pass through it and are processed. In fact, all sensations except smell are processed in the thalamus. Nerve cells related to smell go directly to the cortex without the relay. Some scientists believe that smell has a powerful impact on decision-making because of this fact, and in my experience working with addicts, smells often seem to trigger the worst cravings.

How Your Brain Lies to You

One important function of the brain is to give you accurate information about your surroundings so you can function in the world. Another important brain function is to lie to you. Several medical conditions provide dramatic examples of this. For example, patients with schizophrenia and other psychotic conditions may experience auditory or visual hallucinations. Olfactory hallucinations (where you smell something that isn't there) are common with certain seizure disorders and tumors. People with the psychiatric condition called Capgras syndrome believe that those around them have been replaced by imposters. In de Clérambault's syndrome, you believe that someone is in love with you even though they are not. In delusional parasitosis, you become convinced that you are infested with parasites when you are not. When people have these disorders, no amount of evidence or argument can convince them that they are wrong. In later chapters, you will learn how your brain actually lies to you all the time, even without the presence of mental or physical illness.

My father, who is a cardiologist originally from India, recounted a story to me about a small village where a woman believed she had a frog in her womb. No amount of rationalizing with her worked, and she went from doctor to doctor requesting a treatment. Finally, one physician put her under anesthesia, made a superficial incision in her lower abdomen, then woke her up and showed her a live frog that he had secretly sent his nurse to procure from a local stream, proclaiming she was cured. Everyone thought this was a brilliant solution, and the woman was so grateful to have been cured—that is, until the woman returned to the surgeon two weeks later pointing out that "the frog had babies" and that another surgery was needed. You can't talk someone out of their delusion.

Brain injuries can provide even more dramatic examples of how your brain can lie to you. In some forms of severe epilepsy, the treatment involves severing part of one of the bridges between your left and right brain, called the corpus callosum. When people have this surgery, they can develop split-brain syndrome—the two halves of their brain no longer work together. For example, they are unable to verbally name things that their right brain is observing because their speech center is on the left side of their brain. They will often make up bizarre explanations for this phenomenon (called confabulation, which also occurs with a certain form of alcoholic brain damage called Korsakoff's syndrome). Some strokes can result in a condition called hemineglect, where a person doesn't believe that half of their body belongs to them. These people, when asked to draw a clock face, might only draw half of the clock (the numbers 1–6, for example). Such a person might not be able to move his left arm, which he also is "neglecting." In severe cases, when you pick up his left arm and show it to him and ask him what it is, he might respond "a piece of meat."

Decision-Making and Your Brain

The link between certain regions of your brain and your ability to make sound decisions can indeed be very dramatic. In November 1848, a physician named John Harlow published a case report in the *Boston and Medical Surgical Journal* titled "Passage of an Iron Rod through the Head" about a man named Phineas Gage. Phineas was a twenty-five-year-old married railroad worker in Vermont. On September 13, 1848, Phineas was compacting explosive powder into a boulder using an iron tamping rod that was 3 feet, 7 inches long, 1¼ inches in diameter, and pointed at one end. Phineas was looking away, toward some of his coworkers, when the powder accidentally sparked, and the resulting explosion propelled the rod into his left cheekbone, through the floor of his left eye socket, and out the midline of his skull, landing some thirty feet away.

Phineas was a well-loved guy, and his coworkers immediately ran to his aid. Within minutes he was speaking and was rushed in an oxcart to a local hotel where, with just a little assistance, he climbed a flight of stairs and changed his clothes, all the while with a gaping hole clear through the left frontal lobe of his brain. A mere ninety minutes after the accident, he was examined by Dr. Harlow and found to be doing remarkably well. Over the next few days he was up and about, with no difficulties in speech, motor activity, or sensory abilities. At that point, Harlow was quite amazed that Phineas didn't seem to have anything major wrong with him, even though he had lost a substantial chunk of his brain! The doctor was no doubt wondering: What exactly is the purpose of that part of the brain if you can lose it without any consequences?

Phineas's wife, however, knew better, as she observed that he was never quite the same. Over the next few weeks, months, and years, it became clear that what had changed about Phineas were his choices and his personality. The changes were so dramatic that, twenty years later, Harlow was compelled to publish a follow-up report in the *Bulletin of the Massachusetts Medical Society* detailing the tremendous changes in Phineas resulting from the loss of his orbitofrontal cortex. In Harlow's words:

> His contractors, who regarded him as the most efficient and capable foreman in their employ previous to his injury, considered the change in his mind so marked that they could not give him his place again. He is fitful, irreverent, indulging at times in the grossest profanity (which was not previously his custom), manifesting but little deference for his fellows, impatient of restraint of advice when it conflicts with his desires, at times pertinaciously obstinate, yet capricious and vacillating, devising many plans of future operation, which are no sooner arranged than they are abandoned in turn for others appearing more feasible. In this regard, his mind was radically changed, so decidedly that his friends and acquaintances said he was "no longer Gage."[1]

In other words, Phineas was rude, impulsive, lazy, impatient, and stubborn. He was no longer the man he used to be and could not relate to his coworkers, friends, and family like he once did. Phineas Gage's behavior sounds a lot like how someone might describe an addict. Physicians had known for many years that injuries to the brain could result in problems with movement, speech, sensation, and consciousness. But Phineas's case was the first to show that judgment was also localized to a particular region of the brain. Put another way, when Phineas lost a critical part of his brain, what he wanted and what he chose changed. His friends were absolutely correct: he was "no longer Gage."

When I was a resident physician at Duke, I began a research project examining auditory hallucinations in schizophrenics with a brilliant mentor, Dr. Lawrence Dunn. Our interest was in rapid transcranial magnetic stimulation (rTMS), a technique where a powerful electromagnetic coil that can activate regions of the brain beneath the coil is applied to the scalp. The device was still experimental at that time, and we ordered one from a British company. It sat in U.S. customs for months while we waited for the Food and Drug Administration (FDA) to figure out what it was and approve our paperwork. (Nowadays these devices are common and are used to treat a range of conditions, especially depression.) There is nothing particularly special about the workings of this device. It's simply a copper wire coil wrapped a few thousand times inside a handheld wand with an electrical current running through it. You could probably buy the supplies at Radio Shack and build your own, although I wouldn't recommend it! As any junior scientist knows, an alternating current produces a moving magnetic field that will induce a current in any nearby conductive material. And the axons of neurons are conductive material. So the mere act of holding the rTMS device over a person's head and turning it on actually activates the nerve cells.

As I learned more about this technique (and as I waited for the device to arrive), I became less interested in auditory hallucinations and more fascinated with the research of a neuroscientist named Alvaro Pascual-Leone. Pascual-Leone had published an amazing study that garnered little attention in the media, despite its groundbreaking findings.[2] He asked his subjects to extend their right or left index finger every time they heard a click. It was the subjects' choice whether they wanted to extend their left or their right index finger. He then placed the coil over specific positions on each subject's scalp and carried out the experiment. What he noticed was that the placement of the coil seemed to influence which finger the subjects selected—he was influencing their decisions by magnetically inducing currents in their brains. Holding a device over their heads changed the way they made choices! But even more important, the people whose decisions had been influenced by the coil's placement *had no idea whatsoever that their choices had been affected by the coil.* They just thought they were picking at random.

Once again, as in the case of Phineas Gage, changes in the brain affected choices and desires without the affected people even realizing they were being influenced! Several years later, in 2007, Pascual-Leone and his team were also able to use the rTMS technique to reduce risk-taking behavior in subjects, something that is extremely important when dealing with cravings and addiction.[3]

Over the last ten years or so that I have spent treating people who are prey to their cravings, I've discovered that it is critically important for people to believe they are in control of their actions, that it seems impossible for them to accept that they might be influenced by circumstances beyond their control. Years ago I met an alcoholic who told me, "Dr. Manejwala, every drink I ever took made perfect sense to me *while I was taking it.*"

Nevertheless, what we know about how the brain seeks reward and reinforcement suggests that these influences are mostly *not* under our conscious control. In fact, most of the structures involved in reward and reinforcement (such as food and sex) lie deep within the brain, in what scientists call the subcortical regions. These subcortical areas are not under our conscious control. In response to survival drives (food, sex, sleep), the brain's reward systems activate behaviors associated with strong emotions, such as bulimia and gambling, and using intoxicating substances like alcohol and marijuana. This means that when we engage in activities that are designed to be rewarding because they are integral to our survival, these parts of the brain activate, ensuring that we continue to do what we need to in order to survive (eat) and propagate our species (sex).

Cravings as a Biological Phenomenon

We now have conclusive and overwhelming scientific evidence that cravings are, in part, a biological phenomenon. Here's a recent example. UCLA's (University of California, Los Angeles) Marc Cohen had cigarette smokers perform three tasks: watch a video that induced cigarette cravings, watch a neutral video, or watch no video at all. He and his team instructed the smokers to resist their cravings.

Purely by analyzing the functional brain scans, the team could tell which video the subjects were watching. *Using the same technique, they were able to predict whether or not the subjects were resisting their cravings.*[4] This is another way that functional brain imaging can be used along with certain mathematical tools to essentially "read" a person's mind. It also suggests that the distinction between the mind and the brain is largely an artifice related to our current imperfect understanding of neurobiology and the science of mind.

Of course, cravings are much more than responses to reward and reinforcement. Cravings involve emotions, memories, sense of loss of control, reward, and reinforcement. Each of these primary characteristics of cravings results from the activities in specific regions of our brains. Some cravings appear to be related to reward, others to the pursuit of relief, and still others to obsession.[5] The reward-related cravings may primarily involve the neurotransmitters dopamine and gamma-aminobutyric acid (GABA), the relief-related cravings may involve glutamate, and the obsessive cravings may be more related to serotonin.

But let's review the simplest phenomenon first: the phenomenon of reward. To understand this simple but powerful survival drive, we'll need to explore some basic aspects of the anatomy and biology of the brain.

The Brain's Reward System

Several key regions of the brain are involved when the brain experiences reward. These regions are located along an area of the brain called the median forebrain bundle (MFB). The first is a deep brain structure called the ventral tegmental area (VTA). The VTA, located at the base of the midbrain, consists of many nerve cells, some of which contain dopamine, a neurotransmitter involved in various brain functions, including reward. We'll be talking a lot more about dopamine, which is a catecholamine neurotransmitter, later. Actually, the VTA has been connected to several important brain functions, such as motivation, cognition, and even love. In 2005, Helen Fisher of Rutgers University and her colleagues Arthur Aron from the State University of New York–Stony Brook and Lucy Brown from Albert Einstein College of Medicine published a landmark study on this very subject. Using a technique called functional magnetic resonance imaging (fMRI), the researchers found a correlation between romantic love and intense activity in the right VTA. This research suggests that romantic love, distinct from the sex drive, is closely related to the brain's motivation system. This connection allows people to focus their energies on a particular mate, thus conserving energy and facilitating their ability to select a mate. Many of my own patients have described a feeling of love toward their drug of choice, and this may be due to some overlap between the neurobiology of romantic love and the neurobiology of addiction. Some of the neurons in the VTA will release dopamine only when a reward is greater than expected.

The VTA neurons connect (or project, as neuroscientists like to say) to many brain regions, including the prefrontal cortex (the part of the brain that Phineas Gage lost), the amygdala, and the nucleus accumbens. The "amygdala" (the Greek word for almond, because in humans it is about the size and shape of an almond) is responsible for processing emotions related to survival. In particular,

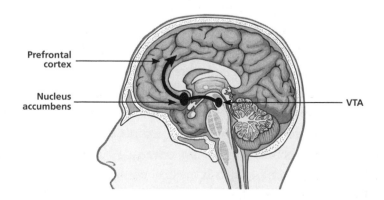

the amygdala lights up in response to intense pleasure, fear, and anger. One particularly important role of the amygdala is to signal the emotional significance of an event. This means that the amygdala decides how intense an emotional reaction should be in response to a particular event. In cravings, this signal is amplified, so that the person's emotional response to the craving is much more than it "should" be. And that increased emotional intensity leads to an amplification in the person's response behaviors as well (for example, drug use, sex, food, or gambling).

The VTA also projects to the nucleus accumbens (NA). One of the most interesting regions of the brain, the nucleus accumbens is responsible in part for pleasure, reward, and, according to some recent research, even joy and laughter. In 1954, James Olds and Peter Milner of McGill University in Montreal published a study that was to become one of the most famous studies in the history of addiction research.[6] This study dramatically transformed our understanding of the brain science of reward and reinforcement. Olds and Milner implanted silver wire electrodes into the brains of fifteen male rats and then measured the effects of stimulating various parts of their brains. (Rat brains are actually remarkably similar to human brains. This was a major ego blow to me when I learned it in medical school.) Their experiments, and many more refinements over the ensuing decades, have demonstrated that when rats are permitted to press a lever that delivers an electrical stimulus to their NA, it is extremely reinforcing. These rats would rather stimulate their NA than eat, to the point where they will die of starvation, just for the chance to press the lever one . . . more . . . time.

Even more interesting is the following: after they have been stimulating their NAs for a while, if the electricity to the experiment is unplugged, something very peculiar happens. First, the rats press the stimulation lever even more intensely and rapidly. This is called an extinction burst and represents the desperation of wanting additional stimulation. Eventually, however, the rat "realizes" that no more stimulation is forthcoming (the electricity has been turned off). You would then expect the rats to give up and press on the lever for the food and begin eating instead. But that's not what happens. Instead, the rats curl up in a corner and die of starvation, in the face of all the food they could want or need! Why would the rats refuse to eat after overstimulating their own NAs?

The answer is critical to our understanding of craving and has to do with a concept neuroscientists call downregulation. When one neuron is communicating with another, a neurotransmitter is released by the first neuron, and it attaches to a protein on the surface of the second neuron, called a receptor, which can be thought of as an antenna. These receptors then change shape as a result, and the second neuron is activated. The outcome is that the first neuron has communicated with the second neuron. The "talking" neuron releases the chemical neurotransmitter (in our case, dopamine), and the "listening" neuron waits for its receptor to be activated by the dopamine. Many of the neurons in the NA have these dopamine receptors and are just waiting to be activated so they can send their signals to other parts of the brain, signals that say, "I'm experiencing reward, and even more than I had expected!"

The number of dopamine receptors that get activated determines the strength of the signal—the intensity of the reward. When these cells are overstimulated (which is what happened to the rats in which Olds and Milner implanted the electrodes), they recognize that with so much dopamine flooding their cells, there is no need to manufacture so many dopamine receptors. As cells like to conserve energy, they will only manufacture dopamine receptors if they need them.

So what explains why the rats curl up in a corner and die once the stimulation to their NA is turned off? The answer is that the number of dopamine receptors has been dramatically reduced, or downregulated. This affects the rat's ability to experience reward. Nothing is rewarding, including food. The reward system is burned out. The rat then dies of starvation. Now the tremendous implications of the classic Olds/Milner experiment become clear. When humans experience overstimulation, as in, for example, cocaine addiction, their NA becomes flooded with dopamine, and the dopamine receptor density decreases (downregulation). Eventually, the addict becomes unable to experience reward or pleasure from anything without the drug.

There have been some fascinating studies about this phenomenon. For example, certain rats have been bred to "prefer" alcohol. In 2004, Dr. Panayotis Thanos and colleagues at the Brookhaven National Laboratory showed that they could use a viral vector to deliver the gene for a specific type of dopamine receptor (D2) into the core of the rat nucleus accumbens and actually affect how much alcohol preferring (and nonalcohol preferring) rats drink for up to twenty days. They basically controlled how much alcohol these animals drank by infecting them with a specific type of genetically altered virus. When I mentioned this book to Thanos, he noted that he had completed a more recent study that showed a similar effect in rat cocaine self-administration. Some very recent optogenetic research has shown similar results with food-seeking behaviors.

The Brain Science of Craving

Over the last ten years, I've been asking drug addicts why they use. The answer is almost universal: "Doc, I wasn't using to get high. I was just trying to feel *normal*." Well, "normal" is complicated, but it's at least in part related to the dopamine receptor density in the nucleus accumbens. Actually, many changes in the brain occur as a result of decreased dopamine activity.[7] One thing is clear: a low dopamine receptor density in the NA feels miserable.

Of course, this is a grossly oversimplified explanation of the brain science of craving. So far we've learned about neurotransmitters that activate or increase activity in the brain. There are also chemicals that inhibit or reduce brain activity. Research shows that the brain's primary inhibitory neurotransmitter, GABA, is involved, as are serotonin, enkephalins (which are related to endorphins), and norepinephrine. One currently popular theory is that intense rewarding behaviors increase serotonin in the hypothalamus, which then activates opiate receptors in the hypothalamus. This results in the release of enkephalins into the dopamine-rich VTA, as I described above. The enkephalins reduce GABA activity in the nucleus accumbens, and that results in an increase in dopamine release in the VTA. A recent small study also showed that people with a certain serotonin transporter genetic variation are much more likely to crave alcohol.[8] Many other studies have shown a relationship between serotonin function in the brain and alcohol use disorders.[9]

Other researchers have shown that injecting GABA-inhibiting substances into a rat's hippocampus (a memory-related structure that is also part of the brain's emotional/behavioral limbic system) causes the rats to drink more alcohol.[10] There are many other hypotheses about how these neurotransmitter pathways operate, but one thing is clear: craving is about much more than just dopamine.[11]

My professional experience confirms that addicts are not simply trying to relive the experience of their first high. That's really only a very small part of the story. Most of the people I work with who struggle with craving aren't seeking reward—they are seeking relief. *The overwhelming biological process in addictive craving is really a complex set of desperate, survival-based drives to feel "normal."*

I mentioned above that some cravings appear to be related to reward, others to the pursuit of relief, and still others to obsession. The reward-related cravings may primarily involve dopamine and GABA; the relief-related cravings may involve the GABA/glutamate balance; and the obsessive cravings may be more related to serotonin. Thus it's possible that naltrexone (an opiate-blocking medication that probably works, in part, through regulating GABA and dopamine) is a better choice for cravings directly related to intense rewards such as gambling. Acamprosate, and even some newer medications such as baclofen (a muscle relaxant that affects GABA), may be better choices for relief-related cravings, the kind of cravings that are distressing or uncomfortable (as they affect the GABA/glutamate balance). We do definitively know that drugs that affect serotonin, such as Prozac (fluoxetine), are better choices for obsessive cravings (such as in obsessive-compulsive disorder [OCD] and bulimia), but seem to show no benefit in "pure" alcoholism.[12]

But feelings alone cannot explain the heartbreaking self-destructive results that cravings produce. They result from actions that are contrary to the person's own health. How are people tricked into taking such actions? That's exactly where the prefrontal cortex comes in. Remember that Phineas's judgments changed when he lost a large chunk of his prefrontal cortex. The neurons in the NA project into many different brain regions. Most of the neurons in the NA release GABA. The prefrontal cortex receives direct and indirect input from other nuclei in the reward system, but it's fair to say that the activity of the prefrontal cortex is directly and largely influenced by the activity of the rest of the brain's reward system.

So just what is the prefrontal cortex that Phineas lost when the rod shot through his skull? What is it responsible for, and how does its function relate to craving? The prefrontal cortex is extraordinarily complex in its roles and functions; entire volumes can (and have) been written on its purposes. However, perhaps the most important reason that you have a prefrontal cortex is to perform what psychologists call executive functions. Executive functions are the components involved in higher-order decision-making. These include planning and executing voluntary actions. This part of your brain is critical to working out what actions you will take, comparing the results you got to what you expected would happen, and changing your behavior in response to that new information. This part of the brain is more complex and developed in humans than in rats. For many reasons, including our more advanced prefrontal cortex, people have the power to make rational decisions that rats cannot. But when our prefrontal cortex is damaged (as Phineas experienced), or is affected by addictions, we fail to make such decisions and often act against our own interests.

One extremely important purpose of the prefrontal cortex is to suppress habitual behavior. Habits are beneficial: they are critical to survival, and they enable us to solve everyday problems and go about our lives without having to think through every decision, which would otherwise result in decision paralysis. However, sometimes people need to act in direct opposition to their habits if they are to achieve their goals; in fact, this capability is critical to the basic act of questioning, and without questions, there can be no choice. One of the most brilliant men I have ever met, and one of my most influential professors, Alec Horniman,[13] is fond of saying, "People are creatures of the habits they created. If most of our behavior is habitual, how do we increase our choice abilities?" Well, to the extent that we can, it's our prefrontal cortex that enables us to do so. Since suppressing habits (until we actually change them) is critical to addressing cravings, we will be hearing a lot more about the healing aspect of behaving contrary to your current habits later.

The prefrontal cortex is involved in the ability to be spontaneous, but also in the ability to suppress spontaneous, impulsive behaviors when they are socially unacceptable or detrimental to meeting our goals. This part of your brain is involved in helping you take initiative, in ensuring that you have a broad array of interests, in shifting your attention *away* from what's comfortable and *toward* what you need to meet your objectives. It makes you feel distress when your actions don't help you achieve your desired goals, so that you'll modify your approach next time. It helps you connect similar experiences together even when they are very unfamiliar to you, so that you can learn from the experiences of others and not just your own. It helps you be flexible and adaptive. Animals such as rats don't have prefrontal cortices that are as developed as ours. They respond to what's right in front of them and are not as able to plan out complex actions as we are. Rats can't decide they are gaining too much weight and then suppress the urge to eat that chocolate cake. They can't think through their daily diet and decide something that they want doesn't fit. You can do those things. In short, you need this complex part of your brain to make good decisions.

Unfortunately, this same part of your brain is also involved in cravings. A recent study proved this point rather dramatically when researchers were able to use rapid transcranial magnetic stimulation (the rTMS technique I described earlier) applied to the prefrontal cortex to temporarily reduce food cravings and improve the ability to resist cravings.[14] More recent (and absolutely fascinating) research has shown that some relapses related to cues and context are mediated by a small subgroup of neurons in the medial prefrontal cortex. A cue or context might be watching a late night commercial for Ben and Jerry's ice cream, for example, and then driving to the 7-Eleven to buy a pint. The researchers were able to inactivate these neurons and prevent context-induced heroin relapse in rats! Other research on humans with damage to this region of the brain suggests that this brain structure is responsible for helping people set an acceptable level of risk. So, some individuals might be willing to go grocery shopping when hungry, for example, because they believe that they are immune to the displays and smells of fattening, sugary foods. This research is extremely exciting because it suggests that the effects of cues and context on addictive behavior may be controlled by a small group of neurons in the prefrontal cortex, which could be a future target for therapies.[15]

When I first heard the story of Phineas Gage in medical school, I thought to myself, "What a lucky guy! He could have completely lost his vision, his motor function, or even his speech. He lost a significant chunk of his brain but managed to keep all the really important stuff and survive." Over the years, as I've learned more about the brain and human behavior, I realized that Phineas actually lost the part of his brain he needed the most. He would likely have done much better with the rest of his life had he lost his vision, his ability to speak, or even his motor abilities.

You won't hear about a case like Phineas's very often; obviously it's an extremely rare event to have a rod shoot through your skull, to survive, and to only lose a specific part of your brain, namely a part of the prefrontal cortex. Yet, in another respect, it's happening every day and all around you. Addictions hijack this critical brain region, and people who suffer from addictions can have severely impaired prefrontal cortices. For many addicts, it would have been better if they had lost their ability to walk, hear, see, or even speak. People usually survive those other types of handicaps, which don't produce the same type of devastation that the pandemic of addiction causes: devastated lives, broken homes, full prisons, advanced medical and psychiatric disease, suicides, and other causes of death. While the metaphor is crude, if addictive conditions weren't so treatable, it might actually (in some cases) be better to have a rod shot through your head.

The Brain's Punishment System

Now that we've learned a bit about the brain's reward system, it's time to look at another brain system—the system responsible for punishment. This system is made up of areas of the brain that are activated in response to fear and punishment, and sometimes this system can override the reward system and actually inhibit rewarding behaviors. Most of these brain regions lie in what scientists called the periventricular system (PVS). Finally, a third system, called the behavioral inhibition system (BIS), was discovered by the brilliant French physician Henri Laborit in the mid-1960s. The BIS is activated when motivation and reward are impossible, but so are avoidance and flight. At this point, the person can no longer experience reward but can also no longer run away from pain and punishment. It's when a person has become chronically stressed and feels helpless to act that the BIS is most active. This system, which is heavily affected by the neurotransmitter serotonin, may be responsible for much of the misery that addicts experience when they cannot experience joy from the reward but are powerless to resist continuing their self-destructive actions. This is especially common as addiction progresses, and the result can be an overwhelming sense of helplessness.

In addition to the powerful brain mechanisms underlying reward and punishment that play a role in craving and addiction, there is also a complex relationship between emotions, memory, and craving. Emotions affect memory, and memories affect emotions. And both memory and emotions affect cravings. Furthermore, cravings themselves affect working memory, especially visuospatial memory, which is a type of memory that records what you see and your orientation to your environment. As examples, visuospatial memory helps you remember and estimate how high your living room ceiling is, or helps you remember how many ceiling fans are in your living room.

A study of ninety-six undergraduates who were craving chocolate showed a definite reduction in their ability to perform certain tasks that require visuospatial memory.[16] In other words, craving actually affected what these students were capable of remembering. Many more studies have shown this type of relationship (in particular, anxiety has been shown to impair working memory, which is the type of memory at work when you are thinking about what you are remembering). The takeaway from these studies is that if you wait to take action until you have a craving, you are already behind the eight ball, because it may be harder to remember what to do. This is why, in later chapters, I emphasize that although there are helpful steps to take when you are craving, the ideal time to address your cravings is when you are *not* actively craving. The time to fix the roof is when it's not raining.

Emotions can profoundly affect cravings. One fascinating study of smokers who had strokes in a part of the brain called the insular cortex (a part of the brain's emotion-regulating limbic system) found that these individuals were much more likely to stop smoking than people who had other types of strokes.[17] This suggests a critical role of the limbic system and emotions in causing tobacco cravings. In particular, stress can both increase cravings and make them much harder to resist. For example, one recent Yale University study showed that smokers under stress were significantly less able to resist their nicotine cravings.[18] Other studies have shown that intense emotions can increase the frequency and intensity of cravings. This is particularly a catch-22 for people who suffer from addiction, because numerous studies also show that emotions are usually all over the map in the early days, weeks, and even months after people stop drinking.[19]

However, avoiding emotions is not the answer, as doing so makes recovery extremely difficult, if not impossible. Some research actually suggests that expressing emotions can diminish cravings; a recent British study of cocaine addicts in rehab, for example, showed that when addicts wrote down their emotions they had fewer cravings (and they were less likely to relapse).[20] My personal experience treating addicts confirms this as well. When people suffer from depression, anxiety, anger and resentment, fear, stress, and grief and loss, their cravings occur more often and are more intense. Also, in my experience, when those emotions are most intense, cravings can be very difficult to resist. At these times, people often succumb to their cravings, which leads to more emotional problems. And, sadly, often the harder they try to resist, the worse the cravings. The solution is not to combat cravings but to outgrow them, and later you'll see exactly how you can do that.

Your brain's systems are much more complex than we have described here. As we'll see in the next chapter, thoughts also affect cravings and cravings affect thoughts; this relationship forms the basis of cognitive theories of cravings. Furthermore, experiences affect not just the neurotransmitters released or the receptor densities, but also the very connections that neurons make (as we'll review in chapter 5). This has particular importance on how behavioral changes affect cravings and addiction, and we'll explore the impact of behaviors on cravings in chapters 5 and 9. The effects that activated receptors have inside nerve cells (on important cell functions such as second messenger systems, transcription modification, and changes in cellular structure and function) are also directly affected by our behaviors and experiences. These changes are important not only in craving, but also in the release from craving. For example, the prefrontal cortex projects glutamate-releasing neurons back to the nucleus accumbens, and (in my opinion) probably forms a key basis for the neurobiology of willingness,[21] spirituality, and recovery.

So now we know enough to answer the question "Is addiction a disease or a choice?" The answer is yes. Addiction is a disease *of* choice.

. . .

3

How Cravings Drive Self-Defeating Behaviors and the Tenacity of Cravings

"Crave for a thing, you will get it. Renounce the craving, the object will follow you by itself."

— SWAMI SIVANANDA

If a craving were just an innocuous thought, you could simply wait for another thought to take its place, think about something else, or distract yourself, and it would pass like any other thought. Some cravings are mild or benign and do pass in just that way. However, most people who struggle with cravings wish that they were just thoughts.[22] In fact, many of the patients I have treated have tricked themselves into believing just that. They assume that they can control them just like any other thought and attempt to focus their attention elsewhere. The problem is, when that doesn't work, they try again. And again. One pop-culture definition of "insanity" is repeating the same behavior and expecting different results. I don't really like that definition, because when the environment or context changes, the same behavior can lead to success where previously it failed. However, people will often repeat the same approach to managing cravings that haven't worked for months or even years. I've seen many patients who died without ever being able to change their harmful and ineffective methods for managing their cravings, chronically laboring under the false assumption that "this time will be different."

In the previous chapter, we learned why someone might repeatedly try the same ineffective solution regardless of the outcome. The brain has powerful mechanisms to drive behavior in a survival-like fashion, and many of these deep-brain-driven impulses and drives are not consistently overcome with the conscious, thinking part of the brain (although sometimes they are in the short term). But the question remains: how do these craving thoughts drive the painful, heartbreaking behaviors that lead to such distress and despair? In this chapter, we'll learn about some of the ways that your brain leads you to draw false conclusions about yourself and your behavior. Specifically, we'll review the various types of distorted conclusions your brain can lead you to and why it does so.

We'll also explore why cravings are so sticky—why the sufferer often believes the craving will last forever unless the urge is satisfied. Of course, this belief is irrational. There is no such thing as a permanent craving; all cravings eventually go away, whether or not we act or *act out* on them. Patients often describe this feeling as if there were an open window, and on the other side is relief, joy, peace, and happiness. The window feels like it is closing, and one thought that sometimes arises is something like "If I don't jump through this window right now, I'll never get another chance. I need to do this right now." So they succumb to their cravings yet again.

False Beliefs

The irrational behaviors that result from cravings can be justified in any number of ways. The ways that your cortex can rationalize acting in self-destructive ways is only limited by your own creativity. These erroneous beliefs are designed to protect your sense of self and the sense that you are in control. Here are some of the excuses I've heard:

- "It will be different this time."

- "I don't care, it's worth it" or "I've changed my mind."
- "I can always do differently next time."
- "I've changed. I can handle this now."
- "I deserve this."
- "I only thought this was a problem, but really it isn't. Lots of people do this without difficulty."

Of course, this is just a sample of possible excuses; there are many more. Deep regions of the brain, inside what is called the subcortex, create the drive; and the cortex, or surface of the brain, furnishes the excuses. This is why you cannot reliably think your way out of cravings (which *can* work sometimes). The thinking, cortical brain can always develop one more plausible, believable, convincing excuse. Just as the worst thing that can happen to a gambling addict in Vegas is not to lose, but to win, the worst thing that can happen to people who suffer from cravings is to successfully think their way out of them. The rare occasions when this strategy works fuels years or even decades of attempts to re-create such success consistently, success that always seems to be forthcoming but never quite arrives.

Members of Alcoholics Anonymous figured this out years ago, when they wrote:

> Once more: The alcoholic at certain times has no effec-
> tive mental defense against the first drink. Except in
> few rare cases, neither he nor any other human being
> can provide such a defense. His defense must come
> from a Higher Power.[23]

This view is not particularly popular in academic circles. In fact, there has been a widening rift between academic and clinical addiction treatment, and much of the gap centers around this disagreement. What's unfortunate is that the core of the argument results primarily from simple miscommunication about Twelve Step terminology. For example, AA members usually use the term "cravings" to describe what happens after they drink, rather than what happens before they drink. The experiences that lead up to their drinking they call mental obsession rather than craving. A close inspection reveals that much (but not all) of the disagreement is over form and terminology rather than substance. I have further explained this debate in the appendix.

There has been seemingly endless debate over the role of cognitive (that is, thinking) therapies such as cognitive-behavioral therapy in managing addictions. These therapies, which are extraordinarily effective for depression, anxiety, and many other psychiatric conditions, work by helping people see where their thinking has been distorted. It turns out that our brains naturally distort the way we evaluate situations, and these biases or distortions provide a significant evolutionary advantage. Basically, we have patterns of thought that enable us to draw conclusions quickly and with limited effort. These patterns also ensure that we focus on the important, central ideas in a problem and limit our focus on irrelevant, distracting noise. For example, if you were about to be attacked by a bear, it is not important for your brain to focus on details in your environment, such as what sort of trees are around you or whether you can hear the sound of birds or smell flowers. Your entire attention focuses on the bear. And if you are later asked details of your environment at the time of the incident, you may think you remember them accurately when, in reality, your brain may have simply filled in erroneous information. That is beneficial for the survival of our species, but not necessarily helpful for historians, who would prefer to have accurate details.

So these distortions help us to be efficient and, in some cases, even to survive. In many other situations, however, these distortions work against us. When that happens, we draw false conclusions from our experiences. This can lead to negative thoughts that drive very unpleasant emotions. Cognitive types of therapy can often help correct this. These highly effective therapies help people, in a guided way, to notice and adjust the way they view their circumstances and thus feel better.

Certainly such techniques can play a helpful role in many cases, especially when problematic behaviors don't rise to the level of addiction, and in some cases even when they do. But most folks with cravings, compulsive behaviors, or even addictions are not able to experience sustained relief with these methods. Although the techniques help, they often fail to complete the job.[24] They need something more.[25]

It would seem logical that the brain cannot ultimately outthink itself, and yet so many people repeatedly try to do just this. The phenomenon is reminiscent of a quote from the 2001 David Mamet film *Heist* with Gene Hackman. In this film, Hackman plays aging gang leader Joe Moore, who pulls off some impressive heists, and here he is being asked how he developed the plan for a particularly complex heist. His explanation is ridiculous and exemplifies the type of absurd belief we are talking about—that the brain could ultimately think its own way completely out of addictive cravings:

D.A. Freccia: "You're a pretty smart fella."

Joe Moore: "Ah, not that smart."

D.A. Freccia: "If you're not that smart, how'd you figure it out?"

Joe Moore: "I tried to imagine a fella smarter than myself. Then I tried to think, 'What would he do?'"

Cravings and Cognitive Bias

"When faced with facts that contradict our beliefs, most of us get busy changing the facts."

— JOHN KENNETH GALBRAITH

A sense of helplessness and loss of control is extraordinarily unacceptable to your brain. Your brain works very hard to avoid experiencing this sense. Feeling out of control and not being able to manage your own circumstances are terrifying experiences. To help avoid this extraordinarily unpleasant sensation, your mind creates the illusion of control, telling you, "I can handle this—this isn't a problem." Your brain also creates the illusion of insight and understanding.[26] All of these powerful psychological processes are designed to protect your ego, your sense of self. They help keep us sane. These processes (some of which are called cognitive biases) also help to make our brains much more efficient. We know that these biases exist from decades of psychological research and experimentation on how people make decisions and form beliefs.

Your brain is designed to reduce how much you need to actively think and remember so that you can perform routine tasks with great efficiency, even at the expense of accuracy. This is important to understanding cravings, because many of your beliefs about cravings may be erroneous but were generated by your mind in its effort to create efficient shortcuts. A neuroscience research group called the RIKEN Brain Institute in Wako-shi, Japan, recently found neurological evidence to confirm this. Akitoshi Ogawa and his colleagues used the functional imaging technique fMRI to scan the brains of people who were using inferential reasoning to make logical conclusions; then they scanned their brains again when the subjects drew illogical conclusions that were the result of various types of cognitive biases.[27] Ogawa found that the same brain regions were activated regardless of whether the person was using cognitive bias or not. There was also some activation of other areas in the brain, probably reflecting the need to access memory in order to complete the tasks. On the basis of this and previous studies, he notes that the human brain is designed to categorize rather than memorize, particularly when it comes to logic-related tasks. This is likely because the brain seeks to be efficient, and this process reduces the cognitive working memory load. Simply put, your brain likes shortcuts even though they sometimes lead to false conclusions; in general, such shortcuts help you become efficient in the things you need to do. Yet this process can lead to some false beliefs about cravings and addiction in people who are experiencing cravings.

Most of the people I've treated for addictions have believed at one time or another that they had some sort of deep insight or understanding of their self-destructive behaviors and as a result knew how to deal with them next time. Often I've advised these people that their plan for dealing with cravings, which is based on their new "insight," is not likely to work. Usually, my advice falls on deaf ears. In many cases, their friends and loved ones are also telling them that their plan is foolhardy. Yet they persist. Why? Why can others see what they cannot? Why are they so convinced that their methods are going to succeed, and that their friends, loved ones, and even their doctor "simply don't understand"?

This is where cognitive biases come in. As noted above, your brain uses these biases to create the illusion of control to protect your ego and to provide more efficient thinking. Sometimes, however, the natural tendency toward efficiency results in false reasoning, and this is directly related to the way your brain uses cognitive bias. Many such biases exist; we'll go over some of the ones that are most active in people who crave.

Confirmation Bias

One such bias is called the confirmation bias. The confirmation bias leads you to naturally accept any evidence that supports your belief and to reject any evidence that goes against it. An absolutely fascinating aspect of this bias is that your susceptibility to it is genetically determined! The confirmation bias is a particularly tenacious bias, because you believe you are reviewing evidence, and you end up with a litany of data supporting your position. As an example, I once advised a patient completing addiction treatment that returning home to live was a very bad idea, as her husband was still drinking and using drugs. Also, she mostly drank at home and quite often with her husband. I thought that some time in a sober house might be helpful, so she could learn and practice a sober lifestyle in a safe environment before attempting a return home. She believed, however, that she had acquired powerful insight into her addiction that would keep her sane. Furthermore, she cited dozens of examples where she had been able to avoid drinking or using drugs around her husband. Of course, her friends and other patients pointed out that there had been hundreds, or even thousands, of times when she couldn't avoid drinking around her husband. Nonetheless, she stubbornly held on to the times when she could and described the times when she did drink as conscious, intentional choices. She went home and was drinking again before nightfall. This same confirmation bias plays a role in helping the compulsive gambler go back to the casino to "reclaim the money they are holding for me" (that is, to recoup his losses).

Hindsight Bias

Another bias I'll frequently see in people who crave is called the hindsight bias. This is a bias that basically allows you to believe that, even though you recently acquired a belief, you really have thought that way for a long time. A more precise description is that when people are asked to recall a former response after having been told the correct response, what they remember tends to drift toward the correct response. Remember, biases serve important roles. They protect your sense of self. It is important for you to believe that you make good decisions, that you are in control, and that you have not been fooled. Protecting that belief is far more important to your brain than seeing the truth. Research shows that people who are more vulnerable to the hindsight bias are often more concerned with their image, social desirability, and need for predictability and control.[28] The hindsight bias helps you protect those beliefs. I will sometimes see patients whose self-destructive behaviors have resulted in destroyed marriages, estranged children, lost jobs, and alienated friends. Sometimes it's drug addiction; other times it's gambling addiction or even eating disorders. When I meet such people and ask them why they engaged in these self-destructive behaviors, they will often tell me, "Doc, I knew what I was doing, I just was:

- slowly trying to kill myself
- dealing with my depression
- coping with marital problems
- self-medicating"

The list goes on . . . but in each case, the stated reason was not their belief at the time they were using or engaging in harmful behavior. Rather, they are retroactively claiming they knew what they were doing the whole time, and because of the nature of these biases, they actually believe that. The hindsight bias is particularly troublesome when it comes to cravings, because research shows that this bias is motivation-independent—motivation alone does not affect vulnerability to the bias.[29] In other words, your motivation to get well does not help clarify your muddy thinking.

The tendency toward hindsight bias sometimes decreases over time, especially when it relates to negative or dangerous information. This is important in cravings, because the further the dangerous behavior or event is in the past, the more likely we are to draw reasonable conclusions about it. (Of course, this is no guarantee that we'll be reasonable about our past behaviors; it's just more likely over time.) This is one reason why, early on, when attempting to reduce and eliminate cravings, it's important to get help from others when making decisions. One study that demonstrates this "hindsight bias decay" was performed by Dr. Britta Renner, a German professor of health psychology.[30] Renner's group asked people what they thought their cholesterol would be just before they were screened (foresight assessment), then gave them feedback on their score and assessed their recall bias. The group that received negative feedback based on their score had a tendency toward hindsight bias, whereas the group with the positive scores and feedback did not. Several weeks later, the hindsight bias actually reversed in the former group, and they tended to assert that they were blindsided by the results. This suggests that in the immediate aftermath of bad news, people tend to exhibit biases that are designed to control fear (hence, hindsight bias), but later on, the drive to control danger overrides this bias and mitigates the effect of hindsight bias.

Asymmetric Insight

Another fascinating bias (or really, set of biases) that is extremely relevant to people who struggle with cravings is called asymmetric insight. First a little background: people who observe another person's behavior often attribute choices and actions to the person's disposition, but individuals themselves tend to chalk it up to situational pressures or context. Research shows that the observers are wrong more often than the individual. That is, making observations about people's dispositions often results in erroneous conclusions. Several other studies have shown that people generally believe that others don't understand them well. At the same time, most believe that they can see things about their peers that their peers cannot see for themselves. We tend to believe that other people cannot see themselves accurately, perhaps because of defensiveness or various biases, but that being an outsider allows us to see our peers as they truly are. However, as noted above, we rarely accept the notion that others can see us better than we see can ourselves.

People tend to believe that they are not very knowable, because their inner thoughts and feelings are complex and not accessible to their peers. Yet at the same time, they tend to believe that others are knowable, because *their* thoughts and feelings can be inferred from their actions. Simply put, people tend to think that the actions and words of others are very revealing. This bias—essentially that we believe we can see others clearly but they can't see us clearly—was brilliantly demonstrated by Princeton University psychologist Emily Pronin and her colleagues with a series of six experiments that confirmed certain aspects of this bias in a groundbreaking paper published in 2001 entitled "You Don't Know Me, But I Know You: The Illusion of Asymmetric Insight."[31] The key observation she made was that "People think they know others better than others know them. People think they know themselves better than others know themselves."

Pronin and her colleagues conducted very elegant experiments that assessed what people think they know about their close friends, how well roommates believe they know themselves and each other, how revealing people believe their own behaviors are compared to that of their peers, how well people believe that they can know someone after a brief meeting, and how "knowable" they think they are compared to their peers when performing certain types of psychological testing.

Their experiments clearly confirmed the existence and extent of the illusion of asymmetric insight. Pronin and her colleagues describe this bias as a special case of *naïve realism*. In other words, we believe we have special insight into the nature of the behavior of others and of ourselves, and that others don't have such insight. As absurd as that sounds when spelled out, several of Pronin's fascinating experiments have confirmed that we really do regularly exhibit this form of naïve realism.

The relevance for people with cravings is that, in my experience, they severely discount other people's suggestions, because "they couldn't know or understand me." As a result, they often trust themselves and discount the suggestions of others, perpetuating the dysfunctional behaviors that either result in or result from cravings. Pronin went on to study how members of groups assess their own group's bias versus an opposing group's bias. In chapter 7, we'll explore how membership in a group enhances trust and how this can be helpful when dealing with cravings. And in chapter 8 we'll discuss a technique for addressing this bias called the Johari window.

To further compound the bias problem, although the evidence is mixed, it does seem that, in general, people tend to attribute successes to themselves and failures to others. Psychologists call this the self-serving bias. This bias can create significant problems for someone who is trying to address cravings. Any of the attribution biases—biases where the credit for something is pointed in the wrong direction—can spell trouble when it comes to addressing cravings, because with all of these behaviors people are sometimes successful in controlling the behavior and sometimes not. If you are unclear why your efforts have succeeded or failed, then any attempt to correct the problem could be unsuccessful. People don't always show a self-serving bias. The late Thomas "Shelley" Duval and Paul Silvia from the University of Southern California have suggested that success and failure attributions are driven by focusing on yourself, being aware of yourself, and believing that you can improve.[32] According to Duval and Silvia, if a person is self-focused and believes he can improve, then success is attributed internally, and failure is also attributed internally; as a result, the bias is limited. In other words, the person would take credit for successes and accept personal responsibility for failures. If the same person believes he can't improve, then there is a tendency to attribute failure externally; in other words, to blame others for their failures. This has significant implications for hope, which we'll discuss in chapter 10.

Blind Spot Bias

Of course, there are hundreds of types of bias, and no one is immune. In fact, one type of bias, often referred to as "blind spot bias" (which is really a form of a broader bias called asymmetry bias), is used to describe people who think of themselves as less biased than others. Some very interesting research from Dr. Joyce Ehrlinger shows that people think they are more likely to exhibit bias in the abstract rather than in specific, defined examples. Additionally, people tend to believe that their personal connection to an issue renders their conclusions more likely to be accurate, but they discount the effect of a personal connection when assessing other people's conclusions.[33] This blind spot bias is particularly dangerous when it comes to cravings, as people who struggle with cravings may severely discount the effect that bias plays in their decision-making; this underestimation can, in my experience, result in prolonged and more intense cycles of craving and acting out, as people simply don't believe that their actions are affected by the cognitive biases we have explored in this chapter.

The Tenacity of Craving

"What is allowed us is disagreeable, what is denied us
causes us intense desire."

— OVID

Many of the people I have worked with over the years point out how stubborn cravings are. They often describe the sense that something has sunk its teeth into them and is not letting go. The harder they tug to try to remove it, the deeper the bite. Many of my patients describe this as wanting what they cannot have. Psychologists refer to our response to perceived constrained freedom as "reactance."

But we don't always want what we can't have. Studies in the late 1970s demonstrated that when heroin addicts were given the medication naltrexone, which blocks the effects of heroin and other opiates, their cravings actually went down. Once the addicts were aware that they couldn't get high, they were less likely to crave! This finding persisted even when they were around other heroin addicts who were actually getting high.[34]

When are we more likely to want what we can't have? In a classic reactance experiment by Paul Cherulnik and Murray Citrin, 180 college students were shown four posters and asked to rank which was their first, second, third, and fourth choice.[35] They were told they would get their first-choice poster. Cherulnik and Citrin measured the students' "locus of control" using a validated scale that established whether their locus of control was internal (they tended to believe that they control their own lives) or external (they tended to believe that their lives were controlled by external factors beyond their own control).

Two days later, they divided the students into three groups: one group was told they lost their third choice because of a shipment problem (impersonal reason). A second group was told that their third-choice poster arrived in limited quantities and that their third choice was removed as an option for them on the basis of personal reasons (an assessment of their scholastic records). Finally, a third group was a control group and was simply asked to re-rate their choices.

The results were fascinating. The students with an internal locus of control showed an increased desire for the unavailable third-choice poster when the reason for elimination was personal. On the other hand, the students with an external locus of control showed an increased desire for the unavailable third-choice poster when the reason for elimination was impersonal. What does this mean, and what does this have to do with cravings?

What it means is that it's not always true that you want what you can't have. This study shows that what you believe about the reason you can't have something affects whether or not you want it. If you believe that the primary power that controls your life is also the primary reason you can't have something, you want it more. This has significant implications when it comes to cravings, because it means that if you can develop a different perspective about why you are experiencing cravings, you may be able to reduce the depth of the bite. In my successful patients who believe in a higher power, when they experience cravings, they don't blame God. They simply describe it as a part of their illness that they can diminish or alleviate by talking with others and practicing their program. By separating the locus of control, they achieve success and a reduction in their desire. We'll explore these concepts further in chapters 7 and 10.

The Vicious Craving Cycle

Thus far in this chapter we've seen how distortions and bias in thinking can lead to problems in how we handle cravings, resulting in more cravings because we cannot see clearly enough to address them. However, there is another force that drives cravings: cravings themselves. To see how this works, consider this example:

Tom is driving home from a particularly hard day of work after successfully quitting smoking for four days. He begins to crave a cigarette again but manages to resist the craving. He notices that his gas tank is down to less than a quarter full. There is enough to get home, but he may not have time tomorrow morning to fill it, so he decides to stop at a gas station. When paying for his gas, he notices the cigarette display. He decides he is only going to have one cigarette, but of course they aren't sold individually. So he purchases a pack with the intention of smoking one and then throwing the rest away. After purchasing the pack, he thinks to himself, "Throwing these away would be a waste of money. I'll just give the rest to my coworker tomorrow who is a smoker." By the time he goes to bed, however, he has smoked the entire pack.

By now, you may be able to see some of the cognitive biases in his thoughts, and there are several. But another force is at play here: the craving itself led to a *behavior* (purchasing a pack of cigarettes and saving them) that was also a setup for further cravings. Most smokers who are attempting to quit will tell you that if there are any cigarettes hidden anywhere, the thought of those cigarettes can be downright overwhelming. The behaviors that result from acting out on cravings are themselves a setup for further cravings. (Tom's case is also a great example of "attentional bias," where the addict preferentially notices the cigarette display and turns his attention away from all the other displays and toward the cigarettes. Several researchers have suggested that there is a relationship between attentional bias and cue-related craving.)

There are countless examples of this phenomenon. I usually tell my patients to delete the contact information from their cell phones of anyone whom they wouldn't contact except to act out on their cravings. Now, if you think about the phone numbers stored in your cell phone, you probably haven't memorized most of them. You rely on your cell phone to find and dial the number for you. But with cravings, these numbers have a funny way of getting into your memory, where it's much harder to "delete" them. The result is even more cravings. The craving leads to a behavior (not just calling a co-conspirator, but focusing on and remembering the number) that ultimately leads to more cravings.

Beyond these superficial examples of how cravings lead to behaviors that drive cravings is a deeper cycle, driven by the emotional consequences of acting out on cravings. This phenomenon was described in 1939 in the book *Alcoholics Anonymous*.

> They are restless, irritable and discontented, unless they can again experience the sense of ease and comfort which comes at once by taking a few drinks—drinks which they see others taking with impunity. After they have succumbed to the desire again, as so many do, and the phenomenon of craving develops, they pass through the well-known stages of a spree, emerging remorseful, with a firm resolution not to drink again. This is repeated over and over, and unless this person can experience an entire psychic change there is very little hope of his recovery.[36]

The sense of remorse and shame that follows acting out addictive behaviors can be powerfully debilitating. No discussion about cravings is complete without addressing shame. As a psychiatrist, I unfortunately know of many cases where a patient's last words were remorse over acting out on a craving of some sort or another. Common sense would suggest that when people engage in self-destructive actions, particularly those that are socially unacceptable "or hurtful to others as well, shame would be common.

Much has been written on the shame that is involved with addictive or self-destructive behaviors, and unfortunately very little of it has been in the academic/research literature, but one thing is clear: shame appears to be extremely common in people who struggle with cravings. John Bradshaw, in his book *Healing the Shame That Binds You*, describes the experience, hypothesizing that acting out on eating disorders is essentially a substitution for shame-bound interpersonal needs. In other words, in these people, the desire to be loved, nurtured, and cared for is unacceptable, and inexorably bound up with shame. Food is therefore substituted. However, as Bradshaw writes:

> Food can never satisfy the longing and as the longing turns into shame, then one eats more to anesthetize the shame. The meta shame, the shame about eating in secret and binging, is a displacement of affect, a transforming of the shame about self into the shame about food.[37]

Although people sometimes use the terms "guilt" and "shame" interchangeably, from a psychological or treatment perspective we think of them quite differently, and most people seem to sense this difference, even if they don't express it. In addiction treatment circles, we view shame as the sense that you are particularly flawed in some fundamental way that renders you bad or unworthy of love. With shame, the core thought is "I am a bad person." On the other hand, guilt is the sense that you've done something wrong. The core thought here is "I've done something I shouldn't have." Guilt is often a healthy emotion, telling us that we need to make things right with someone or that we need to correct our behavior in the future.

However, with shame there are no amends or corrective behaviors that can resolve the feeling that you are bad. In this way of looking at shame and guilt, guilt does not threaten a person's core identity. Shame, however, is devastating to the all-important sense of worth and value that people need in order to navigate their lives with dignity and integrity.

Culturally, our sense of shame has changed over the last few decades. Some groundbreaking work by Thomas Scheff of the University of California–Santa Barbara has demonstrated that Western societies tend to suppress shame. However, in that same research, Scheff also found that the threshold for shame in Western societies has been decreasing.[38] What that means is that we are both more likely to experience shame and more likely to suppress it, which should be considered a recipe for disaster. As the gap between what we experience and what we can express grows, we get sicker.

Sometimes people with addiction are so disconnected from their emotions as a result of acting out that they demonstrate what psychologists call neurotic defenses, such as emotional detachment, rather than overt shame. This appears to be more common in men.[39] In those cases, people who are experiencing shame may actually come across as an "emotional wall." To an observer, they may look as though they aren't experiencing any emotions at all. They may seem unflappable, as if they are numb or immune to situations that would cause most people to experience (and express) profound emotions. It's very easy to look at people who are expressing self-pity or self-loathing and see that they are dealing with shame. It's much more difficult to see the shame behind the tough exterior and detachment of those who seem emotionally numb. In both cases, however, dealing with shame is critical if there is to be any relief.

Because shame is uncomfortable, many people try to avoid it or pretend it isn't there, and psychotherapists are not immune to that either. I've seen many cases where therapists treated shame in a very superficial way, often because of their own discomfort with the topic. At any sign or expression of shame that a person might show, the therapist pulls away, tries to redirect, or glibly explains away the notion. For example, a patient may express a shameful thought or belief (either verbally or nonverbally), and the therapist immediately jumps in and tries to convince the sufferer that it isn't true—that really they are a good person. As a result of this reaction, the patient's experience is not validated, the real issues are avoided, and the shame grows covertly. The original shame is still there, plus now the person feels ashamed for ever having such feelings in the first place.

In my experience supervising therapists, this is much more common than most people realize. Essentially, an unconscious collusion develops between the therapist and the patient to avoid dealing with the issue of shame, and that severely limits any progress. What makes this even more difficult is that if you ask the therapist how the therapy is going, they will often reply that it's going swimmingly. In the meantime, the issues that really need to be resolved aren't even being touched.

In my clinical experience, for many people who suffer from cravings, trauma, addiction, or any number of self-destructive behaviors, shame plays a key role in fueling addiction. Thus, shame seems clinically to be both a contributor to addictive behaviors and a result of addictive behaviors.[40]

And, as we'll explore later, only love can neutralize shame.

* * *

In this chapter, you have learned that your cravings and the resulting behaviors aren't just unpleasant nuisances. They actually can lead to changes in your thoughts and behaviors that make it more likely for you to crave in the future. You've learned that your brain tricks you into accepting false beliefs about yourself, your cravings, and the things you crave. You've seen how tenacious these cravings can be, and you've learned that one of the most powerful toxic elements in the craving cycle is shame. Later, in chapters 6–10, we'll discuss the types of simple actions you can take to neutralize the powerful forces that drive cravings and addictive behaviors. But first, it is important to examine how the various addictive behaviors are similar across the spectrum, how they are different, and how your thoughts and actions can actually change your brain.

. . .

4

Addiction Is Addiction
How Gambling, Food, Sex, Alcohol, and Drug Addiction Are Related

"Just because you got the monkey off your back
does not mean the circus has left town."

— GEORGE CARLIN

The old adage that there is no accounting for taste is only partially true. We do know that powerful genetic factors drive many addictive disorders; the most robust associations are with alcoholism. Decades of research have shown that genetics account for about 40–60 percent of the risk of acquiring alcoholism.[41] Half of the brothers of the first alcoholics in a family have alcoholism, and a quarter of the sisters of the first alcoholics in a family have alcoholism.[42] Adopted twin studies (where identical twins are adopted into separate families) have shown that the increased risk occurs even when the child is raised in a nonalcoholic home.

The brothers and sisters of the first cocaine-dependent person in a family are 1.7 times more likely to have cocaine dependence than the general population. Similarly, the siblings of a marijuana-dependent person are 1.8 times more likely to develop marijuana addiction. With habitual nicotine smokers, the relative risk is also about 1.8. The list goes on, but the bottom line is that genetic risk does play a role in developing chemical addiction. Thus, there is at least some accounting for taste.

Cross-Addiction

Among people who treat addiction, and among communities of recovering alcoholics and addicts, the notion of cross-addiction (being addicted to multiple substances or behaviors) is frequently encountered. Recovering alcoholics and addicts have discovered that the use of intoxicating substances such as painkillers or marijuana increases their risk of relapsing to their drug of choice and can produce dependence "as devastating as dependence on alcohol."[43] And yet it's nearly impossible to completely avoid all mood-altering substances; in surgery and following physical trauma, taking pain medications is often necessary.

In academic circles, cross-addiction is described as the "comorbidity" of addictive disorders. Studies have examined myriad aspects of these comorbidities, looking at a broad range of questions, from "How often do heroin addicts abuse alcohol?" to "How common is cocaine abuse among alcoholics?" and so on. The general consensus is that these disorders often do run together, and many people with addiction will abuse more than one substance. We have known for a long time, for example, that alcohol use increases cigarette cravings.[44]

Similarities in Process and Behavioral Addictions

Research has also shown a link between chemical addictions and so-called process addictions or behavioral addictions (such as compulsive eating, compulsive gambling, compulsive shopping, kleptomania, and sexual addictions). The academic community has not universally accepted these disorders as addictions; for example, they are not generally classified as addictive disorders in the fourth edition (text revision) of the American Psychiatric Association's diagnostic manual.[45] In fact, some of what I refer to as process addiction is currently defined as either obsessive-compulsive disorder (OCD) or impulse control disorder, and for some process addictions there are not yet any widely accepted diagnostic standards. However, from a clinical standpoint (and certainly in my experience), these process addictions exhibit most of the core features of addiction, including craving, tolerance and withdrawal, using more and longer than intended, unsuccessful efforts to control or limit the behaviors, and acting out despite significant, debilitating, and adverse consequences. Furthermore, many studies have shown similar neurobiological changes in process addictions as in chemical addictions, and imaging and genetic studies reveal some similarities as well.

In fact, there is significant overlap between process addictions and chemical addictions. About 6 percent of people with alcohol use disorders also meet criteria for OCD, and over 11 percent of opiate addicts meet criteria for OCD; that's much higher than the general population. Impulse control disorders are also more common among people with addiction, and over a third of patients with OCD also have another impulse control disorder.[46]

From a brain science perspective, although clearly understudied, some similarities emerge between impulse control disorders and substance use disorders. For example, attempting to resist the urges in OCD, the impulses in impulse control disorders, and the cravings in chemical addictions all result in activation of the orbital prefrontal cortex. Furthermore, activation of symptoms in OCD and impulse control disorders, and activation of cravings in chemical addictions all result in increased activity in the striatum—a deep brain structure that also contains the nucleus accumbens, important in addictions. And we learned that these brain regions were involved by studying patients with the imaging technique functional MRI, which can, in real time, tell us what parts of the brain are more active. There are also some brain chemistry similarities that, while not definitive, do suggest some shared processes in these disorders.[47] Critics of this view note that many of these findings also occur in conditions that are clearly not addictive. These critics, therefore, are reluctant to consider these compulsive and impulsive disorders as fundamentally addictive disorders. Nevertheless, while these disorders don't have identical neurobiological processes (nor would we expect them to), they do have some clear similarities, both biologically and, especially, clinically.

As an example, let's look at kleptomania. For years, I have seen a link between compulsive shoplifting, bulimia, and (eventual) benzodiazepine addiction. (Benzodiazepines are antianxiety medications such as Valium, Ativan, and Xanax.) I've treated many women with all three conditions. There isn't very much literature on this triad. I've even spoken with store owners who note that over-the-counter diet pills are a commonly stolen item. When I interview these women, they often tell me that they don't understand why they steal or why they like benzodiazepines, except to say that these behaviors provide "relief." Further investigation sometimes reveals a chain of reactions—the women feel a profound sense of shame that is anesthetized by the sense of control they gain by stealing, which in turn causes guilt that they suppress by bingeing, which leads to shame that they primitively "undo" by vomiting, resulting in distress that they alleviate by benzodiazepine use. You can imagine any permutation of the above. The end result is a complex knot that often defies unraveling.

Research has confirmed some of these connections. For example, immediate family members of kleptomaniacs are more likely to have alcohol use disorders and psychiatric disorders.[48] Jon Grant, from the University of Minnesota, has noted that imaging data supports a link between kleptomania and addiction.[49] He has also pointed out some similarities between chemical addictions and kleptomania in the brain's dopamine and serotonin systems, and has published data that supports using naltrexone—an effective medication in the treatment of alcoholism—to help those with kleptomania.[50]

Gambling addicts also share some characteristics with people who are chemically dependent, including some clinical features and related brain changes. For example, people addicted to gambling show low levels of metabolites of serotonin in their spinal fluid (just as other addicts do). We've previously reviewed the importance of dopamine in the brain's reward pathway and its relationship to chemical addictions. When problem gamblers are given amphetamine, which affects reward-system dopamine, their motivation to gamble increases. For example, the ventromedial prefrontal cortex is involved when drug addicts make decisions about risk and reward. Imaging studies show a reduction in activity in this same region when gambling addicts are presented with gambling cues. In fact, the brain changes that occur with gambling addiction are so similar to what happens during chemical addictions that researchers have proposed that its classification should be changed from an impulse control disorder to an addictive disorder, and I strongly agree.[51] Close (first-degree) relatives of people with drug addiction also have an increased risk of developing gambling problems compared to the general population.[52]

In terms of behavior, gambling addiction seems in many ways to be virtually indistinguishable from chemical addictions. Craving, tolerance, withdrawal, unsuccessful efforts to control the behavior, frequent promises to quit, significant deterioration in the major areas of life function—these and many more characteristics typically seen in chemical addictions are also hallmark features of gambling addiction. When it comes to treatment and recovery, Twelve Step approaches are effective for gambling addicts (just as they are for chemical dependency), and some of the medications used to treat chemical addictions also show some benefit in gambling addicts, most notably the opiate-blocking drug naltrexone.

Similar brain findings have been noted for people who struggle with binge eating. Binge eating involves eating a large amount of food, often to the point of feeling uncomfortably full, and while experiencing a loss of control. Many of the binge-eating patients I have treated describe a trancelike high during the episode and a release from care and worry or a reduction in stress while they are bingeing. Dr. Gene-Jack Wang from the University of Florida found that when obese bingers are compared to obese non-bingers, the binge eaters release more dopamine in the brain's reward pathway. People with obesity also have higher rates of attention deficit disorder (ADD) and Alzheimer's disease, suggesting the possibility of some overlapping brain mechanisms.

Obesity has been linked with smaller cortical brain volumes. Of course, obesity can cause other medical conditions that might be confounding variables, but even in physically and otherwise medically healthy obese people, higher body mass index (BMI) has been associated with lower cognitive functioning.[53] Wang recently released a study in which he and colleagues found reduced prefrontal cortex activity in study participants who had a higher BMI; he was able to correlate those findings with reduced executive functioning and memory.[54] As a reminder, the prefrontal cortex is the part of the brain that was severely damaged in the railroad worker Phineas Gage, resulting in his difficulty with planning and judgment. (See our discussion of Phineas and the prefrontal cortex in chapter 2.) The takeaway here is that obese binge eaters may experience many of the same neurobiological issues as people with chemical addictions, further suggesting that these compulsive overeaters may have a form of addiction.

Finally, it's important to note that cultural factors can influence the expression of all addictions, especially food addictions. For example, some evidence suggests that rice cravings are more common in Asian females.[55] When it comes to overeating and food cravings, it appears that the environment you were raised in, the food you grew up on, and the foods you saw others eating around you may play a role in your specific cravings.

Another behavior with addictive features is compulsive or addictive exercise. Many of the people I've treated who struggle with this also had bulimia or another eating disorder, or they struggled with a profoundly distorted self-image. In the professional athletes I've treated, it can be very difficult to differentiate between healthy behaviors and addictive behaviors, especially when the career itself may have been selected for very unhealthy reasons. (For example, someone with an eating disorder may choose to pursue running to lose weight and act out on the eating disorder.) The people I've helped with this problem often describe experiencing a sense of tolerance; that is, they need to increase the intensity or time spent exercising to achieve the same effect they previously attained with less exercise. They describe irritability when they miss an exercise session and often will tell me (especially once they are "detoxed") that they were exercising specifically to alter their mood or to escape reality. They describe exercise as the most important thing in their lives, and they have usually experienced conflicts with their loved ones over how much and how often they are exercising.[56] Research also shows that compulsive exercisers tend to be independent high achievers with the strong "internal locus of control" that we discussed earlier—they have a strong sense that they can control their life experiences. They are frequently dissatisfied with their lives and their body image, they tend to isolate, and they do not enjoy their free time.[57] The thought of stopping exercise, even for a brief period, is terrifying to them. One researcher of these exercisers enrolled 200 people into a study, but when they were told that the study required them to stop exercising for three days, 178 of participants withdrew, leaving only 22 to complete the study.[58]

Sometimes when I describe this condition to audiences, members will say, "I *wish* I were addicted to exercise!" This reaction is an example of a cognitive bias (which we learned about in chapter 3) called focusing effect. This bias causes people to focus excessively on one aspect of a situation, ignoring others, resulting in decisions that don't achieve their own goals. I'll usually counter by asking something like, "So you'd like to compromise your job, your marriage, lose time with your kids, and develop a sense of life that is so distorted that exercise becomes more important than everyone and everything you love?" Often the person's response will be "Umm ... no. . . . I'd just like to exercise more and not hate it so much."

This also brings up the problem with our pop-culture approach of calling everything addiction: the United States is "addicted" to oil, that woman is "addicted" to lip gloss, my cousin is "addicted" to a certain HBO series. The problem with using "addiction" in this way is that it softens the severity of the term and thereby moderates true addictions in our mind; this also reinforces the types of bias and distortion that allow someone to say, "I wish I were addicted to exercise."

Much like with other addictions and other drivers of the reward pathway, the brain science of exercise implicates dopamine, with mouse and rat studies showing increased dopamine levels in the nucleus accumbens with exercise (think rodents running on a treadmill).[59] Many people with exercise dependence also suffer from eating disorders, and some evidence points to shared neurobiology and hormonal effects between these conditions.[60]

No discussion of craving would be complete without exploring passionate craving. Of course, poets and writers have frequently compared love to addiction. Although "love addiction" or "passion addiction" are not currently scientifically accepted disorders (nor are they very clearly defined), there is little doubt that these conditions do share features with chemical addiction. People with love addiction are addicted to relationships or the feeling of love. They may experience extreme neediness in relationships; they fall in love extremely quickly, are unable to end unhealthy relationships, and spend nearly all of their time fantasizing about their partner, the "love object," or about the relationship. This type of addiction can also produce physical symptoms, as with chemical addiction.[61] For example, euphoria and intoxication-like effects are often experienced when the person is in the presence of the love object, and sleep disturbance, agitation, and withdrawal-like features occur in the absence of the love object. Increasing intensity is often needed to experience relief (tolerance), and the object is pursued at significant, usually self-destructive personal cost. Some of the neurobiological changes that occur in addiction (which we reviewed in chapter 2) also occur in passion, sex, and love, including activation of the dopamine-based mesolimbic reward system.[62] People can even experience an addictive "high" from grieving, which can make it hard to stop grieving. Perhaps you may know someone who seems chronically attached to their grieving and simply cannot stop. As miserable as it is, they continue to grieve. As with the later stages of drug addiction, the act of grieving is not pleasurable, but rather offers some sense of relief. Indeed, intense, enduring grief can stimulate this dopamine pathway, and some experts propose that the rewarding aspect of such grief actually interferes with the successful navigation of the grieving process.[63]

So the body of evidence demonstrating similarities between various addictive disorders is strong and growing. This explains the popularity of Twelve Step approaches for managing behaviors that are not yet medically defined as addictions (Gamblers Anonymous, Sex and Love Addicts Anonymous, Overeaters Anonymous, and many more). Furthermore, the core similarities between various chemical addictions are a key principle of the Narcotics Anonymous (NA) program. The pamphlet *Welcome to Narcotics Anonymous* states:

> It is not important which drugs you used; you're welcome here if you want to stop using. Most addicts experience very similar feelings, and it is in focusing on our similarities, rather than our differences, that we are helpful to one another.[64]

This suggests that the collective experience of NA members—many of whom have managed to stay clean for decades—is that, in general, the similarities are more important than the differences. Of course, it's precisely the diversity of the stories in these fellowships that enables newcomers to connect, to finally hear their own story told by someone else, which then creates the opportunity for them to begin seeing the similarities between themselves and all the other members. These members focus on what has worked for them and are unencumbered by the requirement that interventions be rigorously and academically studied prior to implementing them. In my countless conversations with NA members, I have not gotten the impression that they eschew intellectualism; on the contrary, they simply note that they don't have the luxury of waiting for the scientific community to test their conclusions. They rely on their collective experience to make progress. For example, these members will not wait for the FDA to classify something as a scheduled (abusable) drug before determining they should avoid it, and they won't wait for addictive disorders to be added to diagnostic schedules before taking action to recover from them. Many of these members had figured out, for example, that the sleeping pill Ambien and the pain reliever Ultram were addictive and dangerous to them long before the medical community did. One phrase commonly heard among their membership is "a drug is a drug is a drug." The emphasis on the similarity of various drug addictions is core to their approach. Although there is some controversy about this, and not all Twelve Step adherents consider prescribed medication to be as dangerous, most members acknowledge that the use of intoxicating medications is very risky.

Additionally, most of the better treatment centers addressing process or behavioral addictions emphasize a multipronged approach that includes most of the same techniques used to treat chemical addictions (Twelve Step approaches, cognitive-behavioral methods, medications for chemical addictions that are starting to show some success with process addictions, and so on). Clearly, these disorders are very addiction-like, even if they are not officially classified that way right now. And in all of these conditions, people suffer from intense craving, which is another reason for us to address them together. I believe that while these process or behavioral disorders are different, there are enough core similarities to allow us to explore them together and to use proven methods for addressing the cravings that cut across the diagnostic differences.

Differences in Process and Behavioral Addictions

Nevertheless, there *are* some fascinating differences between addictions that are also worth exploring. For example, people with addiction are prone to developing depression, but in opiate addicts the type of depression is often very different, with more self-criticism, worthlessness, and shame than in non-opiate addicts.[65] One theory for this argues that these addicts initially begin using opiates in order to provide relief from a harsh, tormenting conscience. In these people, success has been identified as a trigger for opiate use, since for these people success, strangely enough, is connected with guilt and shame.[66] Over the last seven years, I have focused on the assessment and treatment of addicted health care professionals and other high achievers, and I have certainly observed this dynamic quite frequently. In this group I've seen a triad of compulsive work, opiate addiction, and perfectionism, which are precisely the opposite traits of what people usually think of when they use the term "alcoholic."

Many other differences have been observed in people who suffer from different addictions—so numerous, in fact, that it isn't entirely accurate to say that addiction is addiction is addiction. There are racial and ethnic differences in how widespread the abuse of various intoxicants is. Certain drugs, like stimulants used in the treatment of attention-deficit/hyperactivity disorder (ADHD), are more commonly abused in young adults than in older adults. High-risk sexual behavior is often seen in adult inhalant abusers and in the gay male methamphetamine-abusing population. Various medical conditions often co-occur with addictions, including HIV, cardiovascular disease, and hepatitis C, and the prevalence of these conditions varies depending on the substance used. There are genetic differences in the probability of developing these addictions, neurochemical differences in which neurotransmitters are affected, and brain differences regarding which regions are affected by different addictive substances and different addictive behaviors. More complex differences exist, too, having to do with the emerging discipline of epigenetics, the study of changes in the expression of your genes that occur without changing your DNA. Many of these effects are due to the impact of the environment on how your genes ultimately become proteins. The typical age of onset, the number and type of other mental illnesses that people with particular addictions tend to develop, the impact on physical and social health, and the response rates to treatment all vary among the numerous addictions. These are just a small number of the types of differences between various addictions. There are countless others.

Even within specific addictions, the conditions themselves are incredibly diverse. For example, alcoholism is a remarkably diverse illness, and there have been many attempts to classify it. Perhaps the most popular division is type 1 versus type 2, where type 1 alcoholics have a later onset, and these two types vary by gender, genetic and environmental influence, and the presence of other psychiatric conditions and personality traits and disorders. Other classifications based on personality and even response rates to treatment have been proposed. One thing is becoming clear about alcoholism: it isn't one disorder, but a spectrum of conditions whose development is influenced in varying degrees by genetics and environment and that vary in terms of their co-occurring psychiatric illnesses, personality structures, age of onset, gender-related factors, and even prognosis. Much ongoing research is committed to clarifying the variations of alcoholism and clinical characteristics of this diverse spectrum of disorders.

There are also certain medically induced cravings that don't seem terribly similar to addictions and may involve different mechanisms. Certain psychiatric medications (such as olanzapine and valproic acid) can produce intense carbohydrate cravings. Iron deficiency can produce cravings for eating clay, ice, or tomatoes. Certain brain tumors and conditions can produce odd or bizarre cravings, and these seem only marginally related to addiction.

Currently, the most popular approaches to addiction treatment treat all addictions the same or, at most, slightly different from each other. This unfortunate approach has been helpful to many, but not all people with addictive disorders. I have visited many centers that pay lip service to individualized treatment, assuring payers and families that the person's care will be individualized, only to learn that this really isn't the case. I have treated some people with very complex addictions (anabolic steroid dependence, or the combination of stimulant addiction and narcolepsy, or any number of other complex problems) that cannot be expected to respond to a cookie-cutter approach. Success can be measured in many ways, but if you look at abstinence at one year after treatment, you will generally find that anywhere from a third to half of patients who completed these treatment programs have relapsed. If we continue to emphasize core components in all addiction treatment (which really is very important), but also further individualize care to address differences, we would surely see some improvements in this metric.[67]

* * *

This book is about the core, addressing what is universal to all addictive processes and compulsive, self-destructive behaviors: craving. In this chapter you have learned how the various conditions that involve cravings, while different in important ways, are remarkably similar. It's this similarity that will enable you to use what you learn in this book to reduce or eliminate your own cravings, and it's the differences that will require you to tailor what you learn to your specific situation. Later, you'll see how you can take specific actions to relieve the burden of your cravings. First, let's see just how your actions, thoughts, and experiences can change the source of your cravings—your brain.

. . .

5

Plasticity
How Thoughts, Actions, and Experiences
Actually Change Your Brain

Though it seems counterintuitive, your brain develops by killing itself. At birth, your brain has billions of nerve cells, but only around half of them survive into adulthood. The overproduction of neurons, and later "pruning" them, is a hallmark feature of brain development in mammals. Many of your neurons are programmed to die if they are not used, in a biological process called "apoptosis" (from the Greek word meaning "a falling off"). This results in greater efficiency, as your brain directs its resources to those connections that are actually needed. There is a popular sentiment that the brain cannot change, but this could not be further from the truth. Your brain is always changing. The real question is how can you direct that change in a favorable way?

Another common misconception is that your brain's development is determined entirely by your genes. We know beyond a shadow of a doubt that this is not true; many decades of research confirm that environmental influences (your relationships, what you eat and are exposed to, what you do) all affect how your brain will turn out. Child development experts and others have directed much attention to figuring out what will give children the best chance at becoming bright and leading happy, fulfilling lives.

It's very easy to feel lost when faced with the dizzying array of suggestions in the media about your brain and your health. Eat more of this, don't eat that. Drink a little. Don't drink at all. Do this type of exercise. Don't do that type of exercise. Further complicating matters is the fact that public health recommendations, while very valuable for the wider population, may not be on target for you.

As with most areas of behavioral science research, there is a gap between what we know helps and what we actually do at a public health level. The reasons for this are many, including political pressures and how some recommendations are perceived that can interfere with how evidence-based approaches are applied at the public health level. For example, in 2010 the U.S. Department of Agriculture (USDA) issued dietary guidelines that dramatically underemphasized the role of meat in a healthy diet, and the response was overwhelming pressure from the beef industry to revisit the issue.

Another great example of the rift between politics and research is the gradual reduction (and, in some cases, elimination) of recess from school schedules. There is a preponderance of evidence pointing to the benefits of recess in children's attention, social interactions, and academic performance.[68] However, numerous competing (including political and, in some cases, legal) pressures have gradually squeezed out the relative time children spend in recess. That is nothing short of tragic.

There are a number of reasons why you might want to consider going beyond public health recommendations to give yourself the best chance at success. Many governmental and other recommendations directed at large populations are designed to be cost efficient. If the importance of your goals outweighs how much someone else thinks you should be willing to pay for them, you might choose to take different steps to improve your health than what is generally recommended. By sticking to the evidence rather than what's popular or in fashion, you can give yourself and your family the best chance at healthy brain development, despite what current governmental or public health recommendations may be. Before we address specific suggestions about how to change your brain, we should review what we know versus what we think might be true.

Part of the trouble in applying the best evidence to your daily practice is that it can be very difficult to discern between "causation" and "correlation." Another way of putting this is that many studies will show a correlation between a behavior and an outcome; it's much more difficult, however, to demonstrate that a particular behavior *causes* a certain outcome. Let's look at an oversimplified example of this. Consider all of the cars at the local shopping mall parking lot. If you measured how clean the cars are (interior and exterior), and then you measured how well the cars were running, you might find a statistical correlation between those two measures. If the local newspaper learns of the research, the headline might read "Cleaner Cars Run Better." Now, while that might be true, it's very unlikely that cleaning your car *causes* it to run better. A more likely explanation may be that cleaner cars are newer and so are more likely to run better, or that owners who clean their cars are more likely to service them appropriately and get the oil changed regularly, and so on. Thus, there's a *correlation* between cleanliness and engine performance, but one isn't causing the other.

I face this issue all the time in my clinical practice. Often patients will bring in some study stating this or that nutritional supplement was associated with weight loss, increased focus and attention, better sleep, improved health, or numerous other health benefits. In many cases, the studies were not *randomized* (there was some bias that determined who got the active treatment and who got the placebo), or they weren't *controlled* (there was nothing to compare the treatment group to), or they weren't *blinded* (so the researchers knew which group got which treatment, which can also affect the results of the study). Occasionally, the studies were based on fewer than ten people! "It's better than nothing," they would sometimes tell me.

Maybe not. A 2010 study published in the *Archives of Internal Medicine* examined the health effects of a daily vitamin on about 40,000 women who were on average sixty-two years old.[69] The participants answered health questionnaires describing their supplement use in 1986, 1997, and 2004. Women who took a multivitamin, B6, iron, or a number of other supplements had a statistically significant *increased* risk of death! As you can imagine, the vitamin and supplement industry responded strongly to these findings, and of course I'm not suggesting that anyone should start or stop taking any supplement without first speaking with their physician. Yet a number of other large studies have failed to show any benefit whatsoever from routine nutritional supplement use. Bear in mind that these chemicals may be very beneficial in treating certain medical conditions or in addressing medical nutritional deficiencies. But the benefits from routine, prevention-oriented use of these supplements have simply not been established. And there is at least some evidence that suggests they may be rather harmful in some cases.

This is the nature of modern research—first, small studies of a treatment show benefit. The other small studies that show no benefit tend not to get published, but the studies that show benefit tend to get published (this is called study publication bias). Then researchers secure funding to conduct larger trials, which may or may not show benefit. In many cases, some of the larger negative studies don't get published either, so consumers are left with the smaller positive studies and will often pursue the treatment "because it's better than nothing" (which may not be the case, as noted above in our vitamin example).

Changing Your Brain

This doesn't mean we can't make suggestions on how to change your brain, but it does mean that we will need to be very discerning about what specifically we suggest. If I suggested a client perform every behavior that had a published study supporting its daily benefit, it would take a client more than twenty-four hours a day just to do them all!

Alcohol Changes the Brain

Of course, the first suggestion to improve your brain is to avoid regularly bathing it in ethanol, which is what happens when we drink alcohol in excess. That's not to say that a little drinking is harmful, but certainly there is a significant interaction between heavy alcohol use and cognitive function. If you have alcoholism, you should, of course, stop drinking altogether. But even if you don't, limiting your alcohol consumption can help your overall health, and, yes, that includes your brain.

This is probably a good point to detour and address the health benefits of alcohol. Several studies have shown that consuming alcohol in moderation is healthful. These studies suggest that consuming a "standard" drink a day (up to two if you're a man) may reduce your risk of dying of a heart attack and lower your risk of having a stroke, developing gallstones, or developing diabetes. These benefits seem most robust in older adults who already have risk factors for developing these diseases, but some research suggests that in younger, healthy people, the risks from alcohol are greater than its benefits. (By the way, a "standard" drink is 12 ounces of beer, 5 ounces of wine, or an ounce-and-a-half of 80-proof distilled spirits. It's *not* whatever fits into the largest glass you own, as many of my patients believe!)

Here are my recommendations based on an exhaustive review of the current research:

1. If you don't drink, don't start drinking for the health benefits. The evidence is not strong enough to recommend that, and there are significant risks to that approach that are not worth taking.

2. If you have a substance use disorder or, really, any addictive disorder, don't consume any intoxicants, including alcohol.

There are many good reasons to make this recommendation.

3. If you do already drink, and do not have a substance use disorder or other addiction, limit your consumption to one standard drink or less per day if you are a woman and two standard drinks per day or less if you are a man.

4. If you already drink more than the moderate amount noted above and struggle to limit your use, talk to your doctor about strategies to address that, and try to employ the approaches described in this book.

Before we explore what actions and experiences can positively impact your brain, we should examine the common belief that alcohol kills brain cells. Just about everyone has heard this statement. Is it really true?

You bet it is. Excessive alcohol use can damage your brain. Nine percent of alcoholics have a clinically diagnosable brain disorder.[70] Between half and three-quarters of people admitted for alcohol detox have cognitive impairment, and alcohol is the second leading cause of dementia, after Alzheimer's disease. Autopsy studies show that alcoholics have dramatically smaller brains that weigh less and have larger ventricles and sulci (cavities and indentations) than non-alcoholics. It's not yet entirely clear how alcohol exerts its toxic effect on nerve cells, but the current evidence points toward two major mechanisms. The first is what scientists call oxidative stress, where alcohol supports the formation of toxic free radicals that damage nerve cells. The other mechanism involves excessive sensitivity of N-methyl-D-aspartate (NMDA) receptors. These receptors, which are the brain's primary excitatory receptors, are known to be toxic when overstimulated. Both mechanisms are probably involved in alcohol's damaging effect on nerve cells.

Some of the reduction in brain volume and mass that occurs with chronic alcoholism is due to a decrease in cell volume, but much of it is a direct result of cell death. These cells that die do not regenerate—they're gone. That said, much of the damage to the brain can be reversed in about six months in many cases. Although science has not yet explained exactly how this reversal occurs, we do know that it is related to an increase in the size of the remaining neurons, an increase in the number of supporting (or "glial") cells, and an increase in the connections between neurons. These changes likely reduce some of the effects of the cells that alcohol has destroyed.[71] However, one thing is clear: alcohol consumption can and does kill brain cells.

What about marijuana (cannabis)? This drug is mired in so much political controversy that it's hard to know what to believe. One group seems to claim it's the cure to everything that ails you, while another seems to insist it will destroy society as we know it. Does marijuana kill brain cells?

Well, probably not. Although a few studies in the 1980s showed some damage when doses were several hundred times a psychoactive dose, in general, cannabis-induced neurotoxicity probably doesn't occur. However, remember what we learned in chapter 2, that your cells don't need to die to do serious damage to your decision-making and ability to function. Cannabis dependence is a real disorder that is characterized by impaired decision-making and major deteriorations in psychological and social well-being. Of course, many people smoke cannabis without any major problems. As with alcohol, there has been an effort to dismiss serious conditions simply because some people can use these substances without adverse effects. Yet many children have suffered significantly as a result of the normalization and dismissive attitudes about cannabis use among their peers and parents. I take no particular stance on the legalization question, except to say that it may turn out to be the best among a number of bad alternatives, if we can also establish an adequate infrastructure and national strategic plan to address prevention, treatment, and ongoing management of the resulting addictive disorders. Without that, it is likely to become an even more serious public health nightmare. More study is needed, particularly in communities that have already legalized it.

So it's clear that drugs affect the brain, in some cases by killing cells and in other cases by triggering more subtle changes in receptor activity, neurotransmitter function, and even the activity of supporting cells. Other evidence, which we reviewed in chapter 2, also points to changes that occur inside the nerve cells in response to genetics and environmental factors. But are there things that *improve* your brain and, ultimately, that can protect you from succumbing to cravings?

In a word, yes. To understand this, we need to explore the term "neuroplasticity." Your brain is known to be plastic. No, that doesn't mean it's made of a moldable resin! Rather, "plastic" in this case means that your brain is not static, that it really can change in response to the environment. The brain you had a year ago is not the same brain you have today. In fact, your brain is constantly changing. This makes sense since *you* are constantly changing too.

Many authors have written hack books trying to justify all sorts of pseudoscientific claims simply by pointing to marginally related brain changes that are seen in imaging or other types of studies. This pseudoscientific approach is so common among authors of popular self-help books and articles that there is actually a term for it: "neuroessentialism." Although there is no precisely agreed-upon definition (and some people consider neuroessentialism to be the view that "you are your brain"), what I mean by neuroessentialism is the unjustified overemphasis on brain-based explanations of behavior and, especially, the tendency to subject brain imaging studies to less scrutiny. Some authors have called this neurorealism, and I am convinced this is a real phenomenon and very common. For the scientific community to accept a drug therapy as valid, often we need multiple studies, randomized, placebo-controlled, occurring at multiple centers and sites, and usually with several hundred participants. We require that the findings show statistical significance.

But I have seen many authors cite tiny or even one-person imaging studies as incontrovertible evidence that a behavior is "hard-wired in your brain."[72] Throughout this book I've been very mindful of the neurorealism fallacy, tempering my conclusions based on the strength of the evidence and not merely because it showed up on a picture of the brain.

Thinking Changes the Brain

These concerns and biases notwithstanding, there is solid evidence that thinking changes your brain. For a great example of this, let's return to the work of neuroscientist Alvaro Pascual-Leone. As we explored in chapter 2, your brain parcels out its real estate differently based on how you use it. For example, a wine-taster might have a larger section of the sensory cortex devoted to his sense of taste. Pascual-Leone used the rTMS (rapid transcranial magnetic stimulation) technique described in chapter 2 to map out how much of the brain was devoted to finger movements in people who were practicing a five-finger piano exercise. Not surprisingly, he found that the parts of the brain devoted to finger movement grew after several days of practice. Days, mind you, not weeks or months. The finger-control function spread from occupying a small area of the brain to taking over a much larger section. But even that is not the most surprising part.

Next, Pascual-Leone had another group of people practice the piano riff *in their minds.* These people held their hands and fingers completely still, but simply *imagined* playing the riff. Amazingly, the rTMS showed that the participants in this group also had significant growth and enlargement in the area of the brain dedicated to finger movement! The mere act of imagining—of thinking— changed the physical properties of the brain.[73] Thinking changes brain matter. Likewise, studies have shown similar brain imaging patterns when psychotherapy works to improve a psychiatric condition as when medications are helpful in those conditions. A recent study comparing twenty-five people with post-traumatic stress disorder (PTSD) to twenty-two controls (a large study for its kind) found that in patients whose PTSD symptoms were worsening, there was greater atrophy (shrinkage) of the brain stem, frontal and temporal lobes.[74] Several other studies on the neurobiological effects of psychological trauma, as well as on other experiences, have demonstrated that experiences, and even the very act of thinking, do in fact change the brain.

So what? No matter what anyone tells you, science is not yet able to use functional imaging to predict responses to behavioral interventions in a consistent, clinically useful way. I know that many addiction treatment centers are ordering PET (positron-emission tomography), SPECT (single-photon emission computerized tomography), and fMRI scans on their patients, and someday very soon these may be helpful in the clinical management of addictions. But one thing is clear: there is not currently (at the time of publication) enough support to justify the routine use of these imaging studies in the management of addictive conditions or craving. Nevertheless, seeing how a behavior affects the brain does somehow make it more "real"—it bolsters the argument that these phenomena are biologically driven. We just have to be careful not to draw unreasonable conclusions about what we see in such studies or assume that the imaging itself has clinical value in the management of people who suffer from cravings or addiction.

On the other hand, we have to be careful not to entirely dismiss the value of brain-behavior research findings. As we learn more about the correlation between behavior change and the brain impact of actions and experiences, we are able to suggest actions and experiences that might be helpful in alleviating some problematic behaviors, including cravings. That's not as far of a stretch as it might sound, because many successful interventions for neurological and psychiatric conditions were developed based on their expected impact on brain function.

The research findings that are key to becoming free from cravings are that thinking changes the brain, actions change the brain, and experiences change the brain. And while your goal is not really to change your brain but rather to change your life, gaining a deeper understanding of how simple actions can change your brain may be helpful as you design your program for healing.

So the verdict is in: thinking clearly changes the brain. There are many examples of brain matter being altered by the act of thinking, whether it's brain changes that result from certain types of psychotherapy[75] or the effects of meditation among Buddhist monks (their brains produce gamma waves during meditation).[76] In a stunning confirmation of "mind over matter," for example, Emory University researcher Helen Mayberg demonstrated that the brain changes that occur when depression is adequately treated by antidepressants also occur when talk therapy is successful. Furthermore, in a University of Wisconsin study of monks selected by the Dalai Lama, it was found that meditation produced persistent, favorable changes in their brain wave activity.

So, certain types of talk therapy heal the brain, and meditation also produces both temporary and persistent changes in the brain. In the next chapter, when I lay out some specific recommendations for dealing with cravings, you will see that I recommend them for people who are distressed by their cravings. What about positive thoughts and emotions? While we know a little bit about the effects of positive emotions on the endocrine system, and there is some brain imaging and brain wave research on the effects of positive thinking, unfortunately such research remains in its infancy (scientists tend to focus more on problems than on successes). For example, we know from both EEG (brain wave) research and functional brain imaging research that positive emotions tend to induce brain activity in the left prefrontal cortex, and negative emotions tend to activate the right prefrontal cortex. One fascinating study actually showed that positive and negative emotions affect decision-making in different ways and that the differences were visible when looking at functional images of the brain (researchers call this the framing effect).[77]

However, even without understanding the brain science of positive emotions and positive thinking, there are good reasons to focus on the positive. The entire discipline of positive psychology is built around the notion that attention to the positive can make a significant difference in people's lives. Happy people function better than unhappy people; they are more productive; and some research even shows that they live longer. Mood research shows that positive emotions improve your ability to think and remember, and to socially engage with others—skills that are pretty important to finding relief from cravings. The mere act of being conscientious, for example, improves your ability to rebound and recover from negative emotions.[78] Research also shows that positive emotions lead to increased resilience, positive thoughts, improved memory and thinking capabilities, and improved social relationships; plus, positive thinking improves emotions, memory, social relationships, and cognitive function. You've probably heard of people who are depressed being in a downward spiral. Well, what I'm describing is an upward spiral, and it is reason alone to do whatever you can to keep your thoughts and emotions focused on the positive as much as you can.

Actions Change the Brain

Actions also very clearly change the brain. Consider, for example, the role of physical fitness among older adults in improving thinking and memory abilities. Many studies (both animal and human) have examined the relationship between physical fitness and the ability to think more clearly. A recent meta-analysis of eighteen studies on this subject showed that physical fitness improved cognitive abilities and, in particular, the effect was strongest on executive function (as we've explained in chapter 3, this brain function is critical in addiction and recovery).[79] There are many other examples of actions that change the brain. The parts of your brain devoted to certain activities change depending on how often they are used. Violinists, for example, have a greater proportion of brain activity devoted to their fingering hand than to their bow hand, and the amount of brain matter dedicated to the fingering hand is much greater in violinists than in non-violinists. So, the complex actions of the fingering hand actually result in alterations in the structure of their brains. Remarkably, this is even true of people who begin learning the violin later in life, which confirms that while it may be easier when you are younger, it's never too late to change and improve your brain through simple actions.

Experiences Change the Brain

In chapter 2, we learned that a rod shot through the brain of Phineas Gage produced significant changes in his judgment and decision-making ability. Strokes and certain diseases can do that too. It's not a stretch to see that various types of physical damage to the brain can produce changes in thoughts, emotions, and behaviors. But can experiences themselves alter brain matter and affect decision-making ability? You bet they can. The most obvious example of this is the brain disease post-traumatic stress disorder (PTSD). People with PTSD (many of whom have never actually been bodily injured, but in some cases were merely threatened with injury) have sustained actual damage to their brains from the experience itself. Combat veterans who develop this condition should be considered wounded warriors. Their prefrontal cortices have reduced blood flow, their hippocampi show structural changes when compared to people who don't have PTSD, and their amygdalae (recall that the amygdala is involved in connecting thoughts with emotions, particularly fear) are overactive. Clearly what they experienced changed their brains, and not just temporarily. In fact, there are some remarkable similarities between people who have PTSD and people who have experienced traumatic brain injury (TBI), that is, physical damage to the brain.

More important, we now also know that healing from PTSD changes the brain in remarkable ways. For example, a recent study showed that when veterans with combat-related PTSD underwent a certain type of therapy called exposure therapy (where veterans are gradually exposed to some of the images and thoughts associated with the trauma in a controlled and safe way), their amygdala activity was suppressed.

Similarly, there is ample evidence that experiences in childhood affect brain development, both on the negative side (poverty, physical abuse, emotional/mental abuse, sexual abuse, neglect) and on the positive side (love, compassion, engagement/interaction). Preverbal children whose mothers speak with them develop language sooner than those whose primary source of language is the television, for example. Early childhood interventions have demonstrated improvements in intelligence and functioning, even decades after the intervention was completed.

There is every reason to believe that it's no different when it comes to cravings. One of the key goals of this book is to help you change your thoughts, actions, and experiences to support your release from cravings and their associated self-destructive behaviors. The actions you take will help you reduce your cravings, improve your behavior, and develop resilience, so you are less vulnerable to stress and other factors that create or intensify cravings. The next chapters describe the specific actions you can take to reduce your cravings and, when you do experience cravings, reduce the chance that you will act on them.

. . .

6

Spirituality and Recovery
How Twelve Step Recovery and Other Spiritual Approaches Reduce Cravings

*"I have treated many hundreds of patients. Among those
in the second half of life—that is to say, over 35—there has not been
one whose problem in the last resort was not that of finding
a religious outlook on life."*

— CARL JUNG

There is a deep connection between religion, spirituality, and addiction. Many major religions prohibit or discourage the use of intoxicating substances. *Spiritus contra Spiritum,* the ancient expression quoted by Carl Jung in his letter to Alcoholics Anonymous cofounder Bill Wilson that relates spirit and alcohol, reflects this connection. Jung points out to Wilson that in Latin the same word is used to describe "both the highest religious experience and the most depraving poison."[80]

On the other hand, many world religions and mystical and spiritual practices involve the use of intoxicating substances or behaviors to attain deeper spiritual connections. Consider the importance of wine in Christianity, tobacco in Native American rituals, or cannabis in the rituals of Hindu saints. I have also seen cases of what might best be described as a sort of religious addiction, where people who

are profoundly miserable seem to require increasing levels of religious participation, giving up nearly everything else that matters to
them, and even attempt to reduce their involvement but cannot, as
they cannot tolerate the process of lessening their obsessive participation. These cases, although exceedingly rare, have had devastating
effects on the sufferers and their families.

Furthermore, many methods for addressing and treating addiction emphasize spiritual, and in some cases, religious devotion. This
is certainly true today with nonreligious Twelve Step fellowships such
as Alcoholics Anonymous and Narcotics Anonymous. There are also
organizations that have purely religious approaches to addiction,
as well as modern hybrid Twelve Step/religious approaches such as
Celebrate Recovery, a Christianity-based approach developed in the
early 1990s. Taken together, these observations confirm that there is
a long-standing and deep connection between religion, spirituality,
and addictive behaviors.

Carl Jung was an early twentieth-century psychiatrist who, like
many singular thinkers, explored some ideas that were clearly
unpopular among his peers. Notably (and, to be sure, grossly oversimplified by me here), he explored the relationship between spirituality and the human psyche. His ideas, along with the methods of
the quasi-religious movement known as the Oxford Group, were
later shown to be instrumental in the birth of the Alcoholics
Anonymous movement. One point that Jung made was that *the
greatest and most fundamental problems of life cannot be solved, only
outgrown.* He pointed out that this type of growth requires a new
level of consciousness and that these problems are usually outgrown
when some new, broader interest appears that causes the original
problem to fade as a person explores this new transcendent direction.

In many ways, this describes the technique that Twelve Step
members have used to "solve" their various problems. Alcoholics,
whose problem on the face of it appears to be the inability to control their drinking, employ a solution that does not, ostensibly, have

anything to do with drinking. They focus on altruism, helpfulness to others, and a broader spiritual aim, and as a result, in a seemingly unrelated vein, their desire to drink fades, much as Jung described. Marc Galanter, professor of psychiatry at New York University and a noted expert on addiction treatment, describes this process as a "relief effect," noting that the manner in which people acquire (through group participation) and attribute spiritually oriented meaning to their experiences can be reinforced by the resulting relief from psychological distress.

How exactly does this work for alcoholics and other addicts, and how can it work for you?

Spirituality, Religion, and Addiction

To answer this question, it may be helpful to understand the difference between spirituality and religion. It's important to note that there is really no agreement on a definition for spirituality. Dr. William Miller from the University of New Mexico–Albuquerque has written extensively on the relationship between religion, spirituality, and addiction. I consider him to be the world's expert on this topic. He notes that in the last few decades, the terms "religion" and "spirituality" have grown further apart from each other. There seems to be a trend, especially among Americans, for people to describe themselves as "spiritual but not religious." This is, interestingly, also a central tenet of the AA approach. Miller points out that, in modern psychological thinking, spirituality seems to be an individual characteristic, akin to personality, and that religion is best described as a social phenomenon defined by membership, belief, and practice.

Several studies reveal that people struggling with addiction have very low levels of spirituality and religiousness and often lack purpose or meaning in life.[81] This is not, of course, a universal finding. Attempts to use religiosity to predict response to addiction treatment have not, for example, been very successful. Furthermore, priests, pastors, and clerics with deep spiritual connections can often suffer from cravings and/or addiction. However, a lower level of spirituality does appear to be more common than not among people seeking treatment for addiction.

The two findings that seem to be most clear, then, are that religious populations have lower rates of addiction and that treatment-seeking addicted populations have lower levels of religiousness and spirituality. What can we infer from these findings? First, that religion has a protective (but not perfectly protective) effect. And second, that a low level of spirituality is a risk factor for the development of addiction. Several of my mentors at Duke (Drs. Keith Meador, Harold Koenig, and Dan Blazer) published a study in 1994 that examined the correlation between religious activity and substance use among almost 3,000 people.[82] They found that, among other things, people who attend church at least weekly are one-third less likely to abuse or be dependent on alcohol. Prayer and religious study were also associated with an over 40 percent reduction in risk for having an alcoholic disorder in the last six months. A Harvard study of a ninety-day residential addiction treatment program that emphasized Kundalini yoga practice in Amritsar, India, found substantial improvements in recovery indicators among patients.[83] Another study of American Muslim college students found that religious activity was protective against drinking, and parental approval was a risk factor for drinking. The incidence of drinking among these American Muslim college students was significantly lower than their non-Muslim peers, but higher than that found in predominantly Muslim countries.[84] Several studies have also found a correlation between affiliation with AA and abstinence.[85]

On the other hand, the impact of religion on substance abuse has not been uniformly positive. Listening to or watching religious programs has been correlated with active alcoholism, and at least one study of intercessory prayer (prayer to God for the benefit of others) demonstrated that alcoholics who were aware that someone was praying for them were actually drinking more (doing worse) at six months, even after controlling for baseline severity.[86]

We haven't yet demonstrated, in rigorous scientific fashion, that spirituality is the mechanism that drives recovery in Twelve Step or any other populations, although the overwhelming belief and experience of those who achieve recovery (that is, abstinence plus improved general wellness) is that spirituality is the essential ingredient. Small studies (including some very good ones)[87] have suggested this, but more work is needed. From a research standpoint, we also still don't know if religious conversion or increasing religious activity reduces the risk for substance abuse or if it enhances the chances of recovery, but certainly that also seems to be the overwhelming experience of many who choose that route to recovery. My experience in treating people who struggle with cravings is that those who pursue spiritual approaches are more successful at achieving a contented, joyous release from cravings than those who don't, but there are always exceptions.

Numerous studies have, however, shown the beneficial impact of Alcoholics Anonymous attendance and participation on sobriety outcomes. Emrick and colleagues conducted a meta-analysis of studies on the effectiveness of AA participation and found that AA attendees are more likely to respond to alcoholism treatment.[88] Another study conducted by Humphreys and colleagues found that among nontreated alcoholics, the frequency of AA participation in the first three years predicted sobriety at year eight.[89] These and many more studies confirm the tremendous beneficial impact of Twelve Step attendance and participation on successful recovery.

It would be foolhardy to discount the experience of thousands of people who have achieved freedom from the compulsion to act out on their cravings by employing spiritual means. I think it's only a matter of time before science catches up with the experiences of these communities of people who have found relief from craving and addiction. In the meantime, why not try what has worked so well for these groups?

I acknowledge that, for some people, the notion of participating in something religious or even spiritual is profoundly unattractive. In my experience, addiction itself can be a risk factor for holding that view. Many who start there shift toward an attraction to spiritual approaches, particularly when they come to the awareness that spirituality is deeply personal and driven by the core notion "to thine own self be true." However, for those who do not prefer traditional approaches, there are other methods that may be helpful, including SMART recovery, which emphasizes self-reliance and self-directed change, and Women for Sobriety (WFS), which emphasizes growth, positivity, love, enthusiasm, and responsibility. Secular Organizations for Sobriety (SOS) defines recovery as an issue separate from religion or spirituality, and strongly de-emphasizes reliance on a "higher power." Sadly, much energy is wasted as proponents of these various approaches debate which is more helpful or attempt to discount the benefits of Twelve Step methods. Another key disadvantage of some of these alternatives is that they seem to be defined by their opposition to or difference from Twelve Step approaches rather than their strengths; in the evolution of these potentially useful movements they haven't yet transcended their definition-by-opposition. Much as third-wave feminism provided an important independence to feminist thought that was missing in the second wave, a similar evolution is needed among these newer recovery programs, and it's my sincere hope that they get there. Nevertheless, in my experience, engagement and retention are the most important variables, so finding a fit, engaging, and participating fully seems to be what really matters.

These methods include some core elements that can be helpful in managing cravings and addictive behaviors. I'll review them now, and you can see if some of them might fit for you.

Strategies for Managing Cravings

Create a Sense of Belonging

Whether it's an Overeaters Anonymous meeting, Weight Watchers, or a neighborhood church, mosque, temple, or synagogue, one powerful driver of positive, healing behaviors is a sense that you belong somewhere, that there is a place for you. Yes, online or virtual communities can be helpful, but in my experience there is no substitute for shoe leather. Get out of the house, get to one of these community gatherings, and participate, participate, participate. Remember that in the religion studies noted previously, it was involvement and participation that made a difference. Similar studies of Twelve Step approaches confirm that mere attendance, while useful, is not nearly as powerful as active participation. Some research does support the theory that active involvement in a program predicts success more than which particular group you join.[90]

Find People with a Similar Problem

It helps if they have solved that problem, but, believe it or not, that may not be essential. A fundamental discovery in the evolution of the Twelve Step process was that its cofounder Bill Wilson was able to stay sober even when the people he was trying to help could not. Of course, if these people have not found a way to release their cravings, it's crucial to try to help them. Bill found that the act of attempting to help others quelled his craving for alcohol and that the value of this experience was independent of the outcome. Of course, if your problem is cocaine addiction, hanging out with active cocaine users is obviously not a good idea, but spending time with people who are in solid recovery from cocaine addiction could be incredibly beneficial. The power of the group is such a strong contributor to success when managing cravings that I've dedicated the entire next chapter to the importance of groups in driving relief, recovery, and freedom from cravings.

Inventory Your Behaviors

Most of the people I've worked with who simply tried to ignore, forget, or distract themselves from self-destructive behaviors have not been successful in achieving relief. The "I'll just do better tomorrow" approach does not work. The idea that "if I binge on food when nobody is looking, it doesn't count" is, of course, preposterous. You still will experience the physical impact of those calories on your body and, for those with eating disorders, the guilt and shame of acting out yet again. Similarly, the psychological and spiritual effects of self-destructive behaviors don't seem to be transitory. You cannot solve these problems or ignore them. You have to outgrow them, and that requires noticing them. Much like an abscess, the wound must be cleaned out if healing is to occur. Many people avoid this process because it's unpleasant or because they fear that wallowing in the past will only drag them down. Of course, there is a difference between noticing and writing down what you did yesterday and sulking over it.

As an example, one approach that has been helpful for my patients who smoke is a tobacco use log. This type of log is actually kept with the tobacco itself—folded around the cigarette pack or attached to the snuff can with a rubber band. The smoker records the time of day, the context (alone, with others, at a restaurant, and so on), and the "need rating," a score from 1 to 3 where 1 is "not very important/would not have missed it" and 3 is "very important/ would have missed it." One log is kept per day, and all the logs are reviewed with a support person just before the scheduled quit date to identify high-risk scenarios and triggers and to develop plans to address them.[91]

Successful dieters have also long known that the process of journaling food intake can make a huge difference in their results. Newer technologies can make this a lot easier; I have patients who have achieved remarkable success by leveraging these innovations (iPhone apps like MyFitnessPal that allow you to scan the barcodes of what you are eating, Wi-Fi scales that track weight and BMI, digital pedometers that integrate with your smart phone, and so on). Many religions emphasize the importance of confession, and Twelve Step programs emphasize the necessity of taking a personal inventory and sharing it with another trustworthy, nonjudgmental person. The bottom line is, if you are doing it and it relates to your addiction or craving, you should seriously consider writing it down and sharing it with someone, which leads me to the next point.

Be Accountable to Someone

If you are attempting in secret to quit smoking, to diet, or to quit drinking, good luck. You are needlessly handicapping yourself and dramatically diminishing your chance of success. There are many reasons why people choose not to involve an accountability partner when setting goals for themselves. The most common ones are embarrassment, shame, and fear. "What if I fail again?" This line of thinking can seriously sabotage recovery efforts, and I've seen cases where people struggle for decades without being able to escape from the effects of this type of distorted thinking. The reality is that you should "fail" as many times as you need to in order to succeed. The secret truth about failure is that it only tells half the story. The fourteenth-century Anatolian cleric Nasrudin is reported to have said that good judgment comes from experience, but experience comes from bad judgments. If you employ the approaches recommended in this book, learn from each of your so-called failures, and modify your approach each time, you will dramatically improve your chances of success. Accountability helps with that process. Laboring blindly or avoiding reality is not likely to produce success.

Another reason people sometimes don't tell others their goals is because they truly believe they can succeed on their own. Often this notion is fueled by the person's success in quitting other behaviors without help, so "why should this be any different?" We've all heard the old joke: "Sure I can quit smoking—I've done it a hundred times." Earlier, in chapter 3, we learned about the various cognitive biases that distort our thinking and lead to false conclusions when evaluating our experience and making choices. These biases can seriously interfere with the sound decision to be accountable. If you are considering trying to quit or controlling your behavior on your own for one of the reasons mentioned above, consider using a complete stranger for accountability. Online communities provide ample opportunity to connect with someone anonymously; while not ideal, when done safely it's a step toward involving others in your recovery process.

Meditate

Several studies have shown a relationship between releasing craving and meditation, particularly a form called mindfulness meditation. These strategies have helped countless individuals reduce stress, pain, and anxiety. This approach has been adapted for cravings with great results. One recent randomized, controlled study of mindfulness-based relapse prevention involving 168 addicted people found a significant impact on craving in the mindfulness group.[92] Another study of 248 addicted patients in a residential treatment setting found that those who used Qigong meditation were more likely to complete treatment and have fewer cravings than those assigned to SMART (Stress Management and Relaxation Training) therapy.[93] Meditation as a stress reduction strategy (remember, stress is directly linked to cravings) has an extremely strong evidence base, and it is core to Twelve Step approaches. If you are new to meditation, an excellent introduction is Jon Kabat-Zinn's work; he recently published *Mindfulness for Beginners: Reclaiming the Present Moment—and Your Life,* and it's a fantastic introduction to mindfulness meditation. I strongly recommend this approach for anyone who is struggling with cravings.

SPIRITUALITY AND RECOVERY

Ask for Help/Be Teachable

In my experience, women certainly do struggle with asking for help, but men often have the hardest time. "Male answer syndrome," while not an official diagnosis, does have some behavioral correlation among several animal species, and while it may have conveyed some selective advantage in the past, it really can interfere with successful recovery. When you think you have the answers, it's hard to hear alternatives. We reviewed this important concept, called confirmation bias, in chapter 3. This is when we focus only on evidence that supports our theory and ignore evidence to the contrary. For both men and women, the bias can prevent learning and being teachable. The most important suggestion, the one that is most likely to help you, may not get the attention it deserves because of the way your brain works to block it out. Talk to others who have successfully addressed your type of craving, asking, "How did you do it?" "What worked and what didn't?" and "Will you help me with this?" Keep asking until you stop your target behavior; then keep asking to further enhance your recovery.

See Things Differently

In Brooke Musterman's wonderful book recounting her experiences working with and for caffeine addicts, she notes the following:

> The key to overcoming reptilian behavior, although very obvious, seemingly simplistic and often the hardest thing is to get out of brainstem mode and start thinking with the higher parts of the brain. There are any number of ways that people can do this. . . . [s]elf talk and what psychologists like to call "reframing" the situation (stepping back, taking an objective look at what is really happening and not what I have blown up in my head are the primary methods I use. . . .[94]

Brooke is not a psychologist or counselor. She's a barista (and a great writer). She simply documented her experiences serving coffee drinks to thousands of caffeine addicts, learned a bit about the reptilian brain (which we explained in detail in chapter 2), and found that a shift in perspective often made the difference between an automatic, reptilian response and a thoughtful, mature, healthy choice. Of course, you can't always see things differently; you can't always step outside of yourself and develop the sense of clarity you need to make healthy, positive decisions. That's why this won't work by itself, in a vacuum. But very often, the difference between giving in to a craving and passing through it unscathed is as simple as reframing the situation, taking a different perspective, taking a deep breath, and simply seeing it differently.

Be Helpful and Practice a Genuine Love for Others

> *"You will learn the full meaning of*
> *'Love thy neighbor as thyself.'"*
>
> — *ALCOHOLICS ANONYMOUS*, P. 153

This is a suggestion that might not seem to make much sense as a strategy for diminishing cravings. You might be thinking, "Sure, being helpful is a great suggestion. Who could be opposed to being helpful? But what does that have to do with cravings?" Well, when it comes to cravings, helpfulness can make an enormous impact. It may be the most important suggestion in this book and deserves close attention and an expanded look.

It turns out that the healing power of love and helpfulness is very real. Furthermore, most so-called self-help groups, as well as most mutual-aid groups (such as AA, NA, or even SOS), emphasize the importance of love and service.

There is significant research to suggest that helping others has numerous health benefits, including increasing the probability of recovery.[95] In my experience, it's a serious mistake to discount the importance of helping others when addressing cravings. In the early history of Alcoholics Anonymous, cofounder Bill Wilson, who was actively trying to help other alcoholics, was able to stay sober while cofounder Dr. Bob Smith had originally been unable to get sober through participation in the Oxford Group. Dr. Bob later attributed his ability to finally get sober to the act of serving others. Self-centeredness, ego, selfishness, and other forms of "obsession" with self are considered by AA members to represent the core spiritual pathology of alcoholism, and working the Twelve Steps and participating in the fellowship are essentially designed to reduce this pathology. A comprehensive review of AA is well beyond the scope of this book, but clearly its successful members have developed an effective strategy for addressing their cravings, and a big part of their success can be directly attributed to the principle of helping others.

Research has also shown significant benefits associated with being helpful even outside the self-help and mutual-help group settings. Stephen Post, Ph.D., a bioethics researcher at Case Western Reserve University, reviewed the evidence in an excellent paper titled "Altruism, Happiness, and Health: It's Good to Be Good."[96] Post, in reviewing the evidence, argues that there may be powerful evolutionary, physiological, and psychological forces at play that result in the benefits of altruism. Post notes that over fifty studies have demonstrated the health, happiness, and even longevity benefits associated with being helpful to others. He reviewed studies spanning various areas including endocrinology, immunology, alcoholism, death and dying, depression, and even the "helper's high" that is experienced with volunteerism. I reviewed these studies as well, and I agree with his conclusion that "when we help others, we help ourselves, with the caveat that we need balance in our lives and should not be overwhelmed."[97] Post recently wrote a fantastic book on this topic (and I strongly recommend you read it) called *The Hidden Gifts of Helping*.[98]

A study of older adults showed that volunteerism has been associated with reduced depression, anxiety, and physical symptoms.[99] Others have connected altruism with an increased will to live, improved self-esteem, greater happiness, and better morale. All of these improvements will be particularly helpful to those who suffer from cravings. Some studies have even shown that givers of help fare even better on these measures than receivers do, confirming the adage that "'tis better to give than receive"! Some of the research on altruism and volunteerism emphasizes that the majority of volunteers do so in a religious context, but further analysis has demonstrated that nonreligious volunteerism produces similar benefits.

Do volunteers actually live longer? Several studies have asked this question, and the results are mixed but generally favor that mortality is reduced by volunteerism or altruism. One study conducted in 1999 by Doug Oman of the University of California at Berkeley looked at several thousand older adults and found that those who volunteered for two or more organizations had a more than 60 percent reduction in all causes of mortality. Oman discovered another result that was particularly surprising: religious attendees had over a 60 percent reduction in mortality as long as they engaged in some (even minimal) level of volunteering! Oman looked at potentially contributing variables as well and found that the lower mortality rates for volunteers could not be fully explained by health habits, physical functioning, or even levels of social support.

A few years later, Oman studied nearly 7,000 California residents, their religious service attendance, and their causes of death over a thirty-year period (from 1965 to 1996). He found that although there was no reduction in external causes of death (such as accidents), mortality from cardiovascular disease, cancer, or digestive and respiratory ailments were significantly lower in people who attended religious services at least once a week.

How exactly does helpfulness help the helper? If it's clear that altruism has a significant benefit on mental and physical health, on longevity, and yes, on cravings, it's not yet completely clear why, although there are several hypotheses. It may, for example, be true that altruism conferred significant evolutionary advantage. If you consider that groups with altruistic members would be more likely to survive harsh environmental pressures than groups without such members, it's easy to see how altruism might have been "selected" for.

Another way that altruism might be biologically adaptive is in focusing the fight-or-flight response. This response, which is very helpful and adaptive under periods of acute stress (by heightening awareness, attention, and the sympathetic nervous system), becomes maladaptive, or harmful, under periods of chronic stress. In short, what helps in the short term can interfere with your ability to deal with longer-term stress. Altruism may reduce the anxiety and stress hormones associated with chronic stress, thus conferring additional advantage in the face of prolonged threat.

Altruism may also exert its protective and beneficial effects by reducing or eliminating the negative, harmful emotions that have been shown to impair health (and drive cravings). Quite a bit of research connects negative emotions such as depressed mood, anxiety, and anger to impaired health outcomes. Worry and stress alone are linked to a variety of adverse health outcomes, including cravings. In Robert Sapolsky's groundbreaking book *Why Zebras Don't Get Ulcers,* he reviews the adverse health effects of stress on addiction, sleep, and illnesses such as cancer and coronary artery disease. Worrying literally makes us sick. Sapolsky argues, as I do here, that spirituality plays a key role in protecting against the negative effects of these destructive emotions.

In addition to the value of being helpful, several studies have examined the relationship between another spiritual dimension, forgiveness, and addictive behaviors. Jon Webb from East Tennessee State University studied 721 college-age problem drinkers in Appalachia and found a favorable relationship between forgiveness, especially self-forgiveness, and drinking and health.[100] In an earlier study, he and his team found a relationship between forgiveness *of others* and mental health among people entering alcohol treatment.[101]

On the other hand, the science is also clear, as Dr. Stephen Post notes in his research, that when caregivers and helpers are consumed or overwhelmed by their helpfulness, it can produce negative results. It's worth mentioning that in my clinical experience, I have seen some people use helping others as a strategy to avoid dealing with their own feelings. For these people, their efforts to help others impair their own satisfaction and the quality of their relationships. Often, they discount their own needs in an avoidant fashion and focus obsessively on others and their needs. One way of understanding these people is that they use other people's dependence to meet their own pseudo-narcissistic need to be helpful. In this view, despite appearing to be helpful, they are actually placing their own needs first. For these people, helpfulness to others can actually be harmful, until they have addressed their core issues of shame and inadequacy that drive their behavior. Some authors have referred to these behaviors as *codependent*. If you think this may be an issue for you, focus on the other suggestions in this book rather than helping others as a cravings strategy until you've made more progress.

The late Viktor Frankl, an Austrian psychiatrist and Holocaust survivor, once wrote, "The facts of our lives are not as important as our attitudes toward them." Most reasonable people would agree that a Holocaust survivor is in a relatively unique position to make such an assertion. Altruism changes our attitude and our perspective. It reduces our stress and counteracts negative emotions such as anger, fear, and sadness. (It's hard to experience anger when expressing unconditional love toward another human being.) Helpfulness is in our genes as well as our hearts. Altruism forms the basis of Twelve Step approaches to recovery and, in my experience, has helped countless sufferers reduce or eliminate their cravings. It represents the very foundation of spiritual approaches to managing cravings.

* * *

Although there is no clear agreement on a definition of spirituality, and various programs have been established to address addiction and cravings, most of the successful methods share some core similarities. To the extent that you can take advantage of the core features I have outlined in this chapter, you should. They have worked for countless people and they can help you too.

• • •

7

You Can't Do It Alone
Why Groups Can Reduce Urges and Improve Behaviors That Individuals Can't

*"We allow our ignorance to prevail upon us and
make us think we can survive alone, alone in patches,
alone in groups, alone in races, even alone in genders."*

— MAYA ANGELOU

So far in this book you have learned about the way your brain influences your decisions and how memories, thoughts, and even the clarity of your judgments can become distorted when you experience cravings. You've learned about the role of cognitive bias in fueling cravings and in preventing you from always making healthy, rational choices about your behavior. And you've learned about the role of spirituality and spiritual approaches in reducing your cravings. However, we've only touched on one of the most powerful influences on reducing or eliminating cravings: the group.

The Power of the Group

There are many examples of the power of the group in supporting you to change your behavior. Fitness experts long ago recognized the tremendous advantage of exercising in groups. Of course, they recognize that there are barriers to this—some people feel self-conscious working out in front of others and are scared they will look stupid, won't be as fit as others in the group, or won't be able to do what's suggested and will make mistakes. Most group exercise instructors are aware of these barriers and work hard to make everyone feel welcome; often they'll meet with you one-on-one to answer any questions, confirm that you can generally go at your own pace, and offer suggestions for alternate exercises if necessary. Why all the effort and emphasis on getting people to exercise in groups? Because groups work. Once barriers are overcome, the group can encourage and create enthusiasm, accountability, and a degree of energy that keeps you motivated. Usually such groups are on a fixed schedule, and this aids in creating *habits*, which are critical to long-term behavioral change. Just being on a shared journey can create a sense of connectedness that can keep you motivated, engaged, and enthusiastic.

The online social networking portal Meetup.com is another great example of the power of groups (and the tremendous role that social media can play in behavior change). This site was created in the wake of 9/11, as its founder recognized the incredible strength that results when people come together around a shared issue, idea, or struggle. Today, Meetup.com users can search for groups in their geographic location based on hobby, interest, shared struggle, career, or nearly anything you can think of. And, if you don't find it there, you can create a group yourself and see who joins. I've worked with many people who used social media, including Meetup, Facebook, and even Twitter, to find like-minded people to connect with. Of course, the usual caveats of safety, security, and sensibility have to be observed whenever meeting anyone in person whom you "met" online. Most of these meetings should occur in public venues, and last names can be avoided. But I've been downright amazed at how people have achieved success by connecting with or forming groups, online and offline, to tackle their individual goals.

Employee assistance programs (EAPs), counselors and therapists, physicians and researchers, social scientists and religious leaders have all harnessed the power of groups to help their stakeholders. In fact, nearly every type of problematic behavior is best addressed by including group work somewhere in the program or plan. For example, a Cochrane analysis of over fifty trials showed that participation in groups approximately doubles the chance of successfully quitting smoking.[102] (The Cochrane collaborative is *the* definitive, independent source for analyzing and digesting medical evidence.)

Groups can convene in a formal therapy setting (where a leader or therapist guides and directs the work) or in a nonprofessional context (such as self-help groups, mutual-help groups, support groups). Some groups may charge for attendance (for example, Weight Watchers) and others may encourage but not require paid membership (like the breastfeeding support group La Leche League). Some groups even discourage meetings (such as Rational Recovery, which encourages members *not* to attend groups but to purchase learning materials to stop drinking, such as a DVD set that costs over $400!). That's one of several reasons why I usually don't recommend that method, although it may work for some.

Groups can be immersive, such as in halfway houses or sober living environments. One specialized type of environment is called a therapeutic community (TC), where people who are struggling with a particular issue live together in a community, and those who are further along in recovery help those who are struggling. These communities gained popularity in England in the 1940s and 1950s, then migrated to the United States in the 1960s and had a particular focus on drug addicts. These and similar communities have helped many people achieve successful recovery from addiction to alcohol and drugs, and even other mental health issues in some cases. I should point out that the methods found in some therapeutic communities can often be rather harsh and, for some, rather shaming. I tend not to recommend the harsher therapeutic communities for anyone struggling with significant shame or for whom the methods may be counterproductive (for example, people with post-traumatic stress disorder). On the other hand, halfway houses, sober living environments, and other recovery-supportive living arrangements can often make the difference between success and failure, and tend to be more encouraging than punitive.

Alternatively, and much more commonly, groups meet on a regular basis (weekly, biweekly, and so on) in a public setting, but the members don't typically live or work together. Twelve Step groups usually meet once or twice a week, but some meet more frequently.

There is much to learn from groups that have helped people to manage and then ultimately eliminate their cravings. The group that is perhaps the best known and most popular in this regard is Alcoholics Anonymous (AA). Since the founding of AA in the mid-1930s, many other Twelve Step fellowships have emerged, including Cocaine Anonymous, Gamblers Anonymous, Overeaters Anonymous, Al-Anon (for those affected by loved ones with alcoholism), and many more.

Research has demonstrated that the social connections AA members form are a powerful contributor to their ability to stay sober.[103] In one study, 655 people seeking treatment for alcoholism were interviewed when they entered treatment and then again one year and three years later. Involvement in AA groups was a significant predictor of sobriety at ninety days, one year, and three years. In fact, increased AA participation between twelve and thirty-six months later significantly increased sobriety at three years. In a similar study, researchers found that when you control for the size of the person's social network, AA contacts predicted abstinence better than non-AA contacts, although non-AA contacts were helpful for other important life outcomes. These results, taken together, tell us that groups in general are important, but that groups of people facing similar problems are particularly important when seeking freedom from cravings and addiction.

How exactly do the social connections developed by Twelve Step members affect their cravings? John Kelly and his colleagues at the

Center for Addiction Medicine at Harvard's Massachusetts General Hospital recently conducted research to answer this very question.[104] Kelly's research focused on over 1,700 people who were enrolled in a randomized controlled study of alcoholism treatment. He and his team assessed these people as they entered treatment, and at three, nine, and fifteen months later, to determine the relationship between Alcoholics Anonymous attendance, social contacts, and sobriety. They concluded that many of the benefits of Alcoholics Anonymous were due to the power of AA attendance to reduce "pro-drinking social ties." Simply put, going to AA helped these people reduce their social contact with and dependence on others who supported their drinking. The researchers also found, to a lesser extent, that the AA-mediated pro-abstinence ties were connected to sobriety as well. In other words, "sticking with the winners"—connecting to people who were able to achieve and maintain recovery from alcoholism— also contributed to a person's abstinence.

So, part of the beneficial effects of groups on urges and cravings appears to be related to reducing contact with people who support addictive and craving-related behavior. An oft-heard adage in the addiction recovery community is "If you hang out in a barbershop long enough, pretty soon you're gonna get a haircut." One of my patients was trying to lose weight but always stopped at a Dunkin' Donuts on the way to work because he preferred their coffee over that of the other coffee joints. He thought he'd be immune to the sights and smells of the doughnuts. (You'll learn more about that sense of immunity and what to do about it in the next chapter.) And for a while he was able to avoid buying a doughnut, but he eventually found himself unable to resist them. The coffee might not be as good, but had he stopped by the coffee shop next to the health club, where other fitness-minded people were getting their morning coffee, he might have had better luck. To the extent you can, finding and connecting with people who support your recovery-oriented behaviors will go a long way toward helping your recovery, as will reducing your social contact with those who support the addictive, self-destructive, or craving behaviors.

A word about persistence when it comes to groups: one potentially unfortunate fact about groups is that they are composed of people—ordinary human beings, with all their foibles, quirks, and defects. You may attend a Twelve Step group, support group, educational group, or even a professional therapy group where you simply don't like or agree with what you hear. In some cases, what someone says in the group, or even says directly to you, may seem entirely wrong or even downright offensive. In my experience, it's important not to quit or give up when this happens. If your problem is serious, I'd recommend attending at least a dozen different meetings before abandoning a particular type of group. If you include travel time, for most people, this would mean spending about twenty hours attempting a particular type of group option. I also recommend you spend the vast majority of your time listening rather than talking at meetings. If you find yourself objecting to what you hear, discuss it with those you meet there (after the meeting ends), but also with your friends or others whom you trust. In particular, a counselor or therapist can help you evaluate ideas that you may have gathered at the group.

I've also observed time and again that those who are most successful look for similarities with others when they attend groups, rather than differences. Years ago I had a patient who did not feel like he was connecting well with people at his Overeaters Anonymous group, but his eating habits were destroying his life and relationships, and even threatening his occupation. "All of those people had problems their whole life . . . mine just started two years ago," he claimed. It's actually very common when people are facing serious behavior change for their brains to generate objections, some of which may seem trivial to an outside observer. After all, who really cares when the problem started? If you are about to lose your job and family as a result of your behavior, perhaps you'd better find a way to use the group, even if your experience is different. I advised this patient to attend several more times and instead look for the similarities and make a mental note (or even go home and jot it down) when he heard something he *did* relate to. I suggested he focus on how he *behaved* like the others, how he *thought* like the others, and how he *felt* like the others felt. That suggestion did the trick, and he is still in active recovery today. When you attend these groups, look for the similarities between yourself and others in your behaviors, thoughts, and feelings. Note them, focus on them, jot them down, and discuss them with people you trust. This will help you overcome objections and more effectively harness the power of the group. Remember, in most cases, you should do everything in your power to involve groups in your efforts to combat cravings.

Family

There is one very special type of group that often influences people with cravings more than any other: family. Most people who treat addictions and cravings in general recognize that the problems are rarely restricted to the person himself; others are always affected. Because of the nature of addiction, the person suffering from cravings may not be aware of how his behavior is affecting others, but almost universally, the scope of the effect from cravings and addiction is broader than it seems. As we mentioned earlier, for some addictions, genetics itself plays a role in the problematic behavior, perpetuating across generations. Similarly, some self-destructive tendencies can be passed on by generations of dysfunction in families. Many programs and systems have emerged to address the family effects of addiction and related behaviors. Perhaps the most well-known of these is Al-Anon Family Groups, a Twelve Step fellowship that helps friends and family of alcoholics find understanding, support, healing, and recovery.

Interventions to address self-destructive, craving-related behaviors are much less effective if they are targeted to the person alone;

the benefits increase dramatically if social supports are included. In many (but not all) cases, this is the family. If the idea of involving your family in your problem is terrifying, don't fret: you are not alone. For many who struggle with cravings of various kinds, family relationships can be uncomfortable, unhealthy, and in some cases even toxic. If you have family that is willing to help, often the most difficult barriers are the pride and ego that prevent you from simply asking for assistance. Perhaps you believe you have already put your family through enough. Maybe so, but wouldn't success be the best gift you could give them? In other cases, family relationships are so toxic and unsafe that family members shouldn't be involved, especially in early recovery. This is always true in cases involving active abuse (physical, mental, emotional, or sexual). If you aren't sure when or whether to involve your family in your recovery journey, seek out a professional to help you sort it out. If you can do so safely, and in a manner that supports your recovery, involving others and leveraging the power of family may be your most powerful tool in addressing cravings.

How Support Networks Can Help

One technique for tapping into the strength of social supports, community, and family in addressing cravings is called community reinforcement and family training, or CRAFT. CRAFT is an evidence-based approach to engaging concerned significant others and social supports in helping a person achieve and maintain recovery. This method involves training family and other support people on how to communicate with their loved ones in ways that support and emphasize positive, constructive change. A recent meta-analysis of four randomized controlled trials of CRAFT demonstrated remarkable success in engaging people with addiction in treatment.[105] And staying engaged is one of the strongest predictors we have of the successful treatment of addictive disorders. These trials and much of the published literature on family interventions heavily underscore the observation that family and social networks play a tremendous role in supporting (or hindering) people who seek to find freedom from cravings and self-destructive behaviors.

Another scientifically validated method of addressing substance use disorders is called network therapy (NT). NT was developed by Marc Galanter at New York University and is a technique in substance abuse rehabilitation in which select family members and friends are enlisted to provide ongoing support and to promote attitude and behavior change.[106] In this method of treatment, the people in the addict's network are serving as an extension of the therapist and can be thought of as a team that is focused on helping the person get and stay well. Network therapy is highly compatible with other methods, and many participants also engage in Twelve Step programs while undergoing the therapy. I'm a very strong believer in network therapy in the treatment of addiction, and I've seen many people achieve recovery using these principles. The evidence to support this type of therapy is extremely strong, and the entire program is based on the fundamental observation that the network can do what the individual cannot.

What to Look for in a Group

The group can be either the most positive influence in helping you manage your own cravings or the most destructive force you can encounter. What characteristics are most helpful in finding a group or team to help you with your cravings? What should you look for as you attempt to find or create a group to help you deal with your cravings?

I believe in the value of "going to any lengths to get well." But the reality is that if your group isn't convenient, it will be much easier for you to find an excuse not to go. Of course, sometimes the support group that is closest to your work or your home is not the one that works best for you; maybe you identify better with people at a group that is farther away or one that meets at an inconvenient time.

The most important thing is that you go, but the more convenient you can make it, the better. I usually recommend putting meetings in your calendar, rearranging commitments to ensure you have the time to get to the group, and having an accountability partner to whom you can commit to attendance. Sometimes it's as simple as committing to your best friend that you are going to go to the quit-smoking group at the local church every Wednesday for the next six weeks. Look at the dates, times, and locations of groups and begin by selecting groups that are the easiest for you to commit to. Do everything in your power to make it easier to go.

Also, look for groups that are welcoming. Do they greet you at the door? Do they say hello? Are members available to speak with you before and after the group? Are there printed materials for you to review between visits? Is there a phone or email list of members who are willing to help you? Can the members of this group suggest other groups that might be helpful? Which ones seem the best to them? Word of mouth is often the best way to find the groups that are most welcoming and focused on helping members get and stay well.

As I noted above, no group is perfect because no person is perfect. You are not likely to find a group that fits all of your criteria. You may, at times, find that your objections and excuses for not attending a particular group may start to pile up. That's usually when it's important to stick it out and go anyway. In most cases, going to a mediocre group is still better than trying to handle cravings on your own.

Once you find a group, how do you use it most effectively? Although it may feel socially awkward, I recommend arriving early and leaving late. Unlike a social cocktail party, where it may be appropriate or even helpful to arrive late, it may be very hard to connect adequately with group members if you do that. Much of the helpful discussion may be occurring before the group even starts;

plus, it's an opportunity to discuss any questions, concerns, or even reservations you may have about the group on a one-on-one basis with another member or, if the group is professionally led, with the instructor. For example, if it's your first time to a spin class at the gym, going early can give the instructor or another member a chance to make sure your bike adjustments are a good fit for you.

I also recommend that you "be a joiner." It is extremely tempting to sit by yourself, leave as soon as the meeting ends, not talk to people, and generally keep to yourself. If you do that, you may be discarding many of the effective components of groups. Consider striking up a conversation, asking questions, or even just going up to a group of people chatting to listen in or participate in their conversation. Although difficult at first, the results can be very rewarding. Most successful group participants are people who really *joined*, rather than simply attended.

If the self-help or support group norms permit it, stay in touch with members between groups. In some settings this may not be appropriate. You'll generally know it's okay if the self-help or support group keeps a phone list or membership list. If it's a professional group (therapy group, for example), you can ask the group leader what's appropriate. Try to extend the power of the group beyond its sixty minutes (or whatever duration it is). Do that by staying connected with members between meetings, if it's the group norm to do so.

Finally, follow suggestions, especially from people who have been successful in overcoming a problem that is similar to yours. If someone suggests you call two people on the phone list, do it. If someone suggests you join the group for dinner at the diner afterward, do it. If someone suggests you obtain a sponsor (as is common in Twelve Step meetings) or read a particular book, do it. If someone suggests another meeting, attend it. If you go to an Overeaters Anonymous meeting and they suggest you go grocery shopping on a full stomach and take a friend with whom you can be accountable, then do that. That said, use your judgment and don't do anything that feels unsafe or inappropriate, but in general you want to harvest the successes of others so you can make them your own. One important way of doing that is to ask them how they succeeded and then follow those recommendations.

Groups are extraordinarily effective in helping people deal with their cravings, and in most cases, participating in a group that is focused on your particular craving is much more effective than trying to address your craving by yourself or just with a counselor. Find groups, join them, and use them.

. . .

8

The Naïve Perception of Immunity

"Where ignorance is our master, there is no possibility of real peace."
— DALAI LAMA

An unfortunately common but sad situation familiar to anyone who has ever worked in an addiction treatment center is when someone leaves treatment prematurely, believing they are cured and will never drink or use drugs again. One of the best examples of this was a man I treated several years ago whom I'll call "Jim." Jim, who was a sixty-something physician, arrived in residential addiction treatment for alcoholism as a result of pressure from his two adult children and his grandchildren. Jim was not the sort of person who bowed to pressure from anyone, but when his granddaughter read him a letter describing the impact his drinking had on their relationship, he knew he needed help. Although Jim was initially reluctant to get help, once he arrived in treatment he described the choice to get treatment as one he had been thinking about for a long time and that he just needed the right excuse to find the time. It was so important to his brain to experience a sense of control that his recollection became distorted and created the story that entering treatment was his idea all along. This is very common and is an example of the hindsight bias we discussed in chapter 3.

After some time getting familiar with his peers, his counselor, and me, he started to develop some trust in us and revealed that, in fact, he had made numerous efforts to decrease or stop his drinking. These attempts would usually last a few days or weeks before he invariably started drinking again. He described strategies such as promising himself he wouldn't drink, staying at work later into the evenings to avoid going to the liquor store, switching to non-alcoholic beer, even taking self-prescribed Antabuse, a drug that makes you sick if you drink while taking it. (The adage "physician, heal thyself" is usually *not* a good idea, especially when it comes to self-prescribing.) He admitted to me that, truth be told, he knew he couldn't stop. My staff believed he was beginning to make some progress and look at how he might reduce his risk of relapse when, all of a sudden, Jim announced to the group that he now understood alcoholism and would "never drink again." He described a sense of profound insight into his alcohol use and the reasons why he drank. He was certain that he had changed substantially, ensuring he would remain sober. He dismissed the experience of his peers in rehab who explained that they, too, had believed at times that acquiring some insight and making different plans would be sufficient to avert relapse.

Jim planned to leave treatment immediately. All attempts to convince him otherwise were unsuccessful. His family made arrangements for his continued stay, with pet care and coverage at his office, but he was very insistent, calling a cab to take him home. He wouldn't even stay for one more day to reflect on what everyone explained to him was an impulsive decision. Not surprisingly, his family was very upset about this, and when he returned home he started drinking again within a week. When he finally returned to treatment two weeks later, he told me, "I'm not sure what happened, but this time I'm *really* not ever going to drink again." Within a week, he had left treatment again. You can guess the outcome.

Similarly, I have worked with countless people who have allowed themselves to be exposed to situations that undermine their goals and lead them back to their cravings and unwanted behaviors.

In so many cases, people who suffer from cravings simply don't believe they will be affected; they believe they have the willpower to withstand the environmental threats ("triggers" in the addiction treatment-speak). *They think they are immune.* Whether it's the committed dieter who thinks a walk through the mall is safe on an empty stomach (it's the food court that got him), or the compulsive gambler who takes a trip to Vegas "just to see the shows," people who mean well often fail and don't know why.

The three examples I've given above are situations that are obviously risky, and you might be surprised that anyone could be so easily fooled. But the truth of the matter is that *everyone* who experiences the kinds of cravings we are talking about has been fooled, even if it's been in more subtle ways. The brain tricks us into believing we're immune—that we'll be okay, this time will be different, we've finally figured it out, we just needed to be more committed, and this time we really are going to put our minds to it. Our brains work very hard to find some singular defect in our prior strategies, and then we focus only on those defects to the exclusion of all else. It's like buying a used car and finding out too late that the transmission is shot and then *only inspecting the transmission* while shopping for the next used car. The focus is on addressing historical problems and defects, while completely dismissing the risk associated with potential or future threats to recovery. Sadly, often what happens when people experience limited success is that they stop trying; they do just enough, which turns out later to be not nearly enough. And who could blame them? Making this type of change is hard work and often uncomfortable. Most people want to experience such discomfort as little as possible.

As if that weren't enough, people usually don't know what they need to do in order to break free of the vicious cycle of cravings. Instead of using the types of suggestions found in this book—such as asking others for help, finding people you can trust and sharing your secrets, joining and participating in groups, connecting with spirituality, practicing helpfulness and altruism, and all the other suggestions you are finding here—they will often direct their energy and efforts toward actions that will do little to alter the course of their cravings and subsequent behavior. There are many examples of this. I've seen countless people struggling with cravings for food who stocked their cabinets with low-calorie snacks only to find themselves eating dozens of the packages at a time. I've worked with many people who believed that the latest fitness gadget they saw on TV would finally motivate them to exercise. I've met hundreds of people who wanted to stop smoking and discarded their cigarettes, but not their lighters and ashtrays. I've helped hundreds of alcoholics who didn't want to give up the investment in their wine cellars. In these cases, and many more, an unwillingness to change perspective has led to heartbreaking results: a relapse and return to the very behaviors that they've been trying so desperately to avoid.

The Johari Window

We can be blind in numerous ways to the things that really matter with cravings and thus begin to believe, erroneously, that we are immune. To help you understand this important idea, we're going to review a concept called the Johari window. The Johari window is a tool developed by two psychologists in the mid-1950s and describes a way of looking at ourselves based on what we know, what we hide, what we can't see, and what nobody can see. As you look at the diagram, think of everything that is true about you. Think of all of your traits, interests, hobbies, personality characteristics, struggles, strengths, and weaknesses. Now, among all of those things that you know about yourself, the things that others know about you belong in the first or "open" quadrant. While not all of your friends know these things about you, the things in this quadrant are known to you and to some of the people you know. It could be that they are people who are close to you, or maybe friends or loved ones whom you trust. I sometimes call this first quadrant the transparent quadrant, because it tends to include facts about you that are more easily known by others.

	Known to Self	Not Known to Self
Known to Others	1. Open	3. Blind
Not Known to Others	2. Secret /Hidden	4. Unknown

The things that you know about yourself but others don't know belong in the second "secret" or "hidden" quadrant. Sharing some of what's in the second quadrant can be very frightening. Self-disclosure of this sort is, of course, emotionally risky. What do I mean by "emotionally risky"? I mean that if you share these secrets, people might criticize you, shun you, or not want anything to do with you when you tell them about these parts of you. You could get your feelings hurt. Actually, you *will* get your feelings hurt. That's why it is so important to pick the right people to be open with and to constantly evaluate the relationships to make sure they are safe and loving enough to risk this sort of disclosure. This is *not* a recommendation to go and share your darkest secrets with the world. But at the right time, and in the right context and with the right people, taking these types of risks is absolutely essential to our growth. Start slowly and take it easy. You'll know when it's right if you listen to your inner voice, and you can do a little at a time to try it on for size. This process is exactly how we grow emotionally and become more mature in our response to life and its opportunities and challenges.

By the way, this type of self-disclosure is also the essence of being tough. Despite what you see in the movies and on TV, toughness does *not* mean holding back your emotions and being an impenetrable stone wall. That would be the opposite of courageous: the total avoidance of emotional risk.

Rather, toughness is about seeking the right relationships, where vulnerability and openness can be risked. It means being willing to experience pain when it's the right time. It's very easy to become falsely convinced that being tough means hiding emotionally.

This sort of deception is remarkably powerful and seductive, and a constant battle when it comes to craving. It tricks you into believing that your truth is not strong enough or worthy enough to share. Truth, however, is tough. That is its nature. Supreme Court justice Oliver Wendell Holmes Jr. said it best: "Truth is tough. It will not break, like a bubble, at the touch; nay, you may kick it about all day like a football, and it will be round and full at evening." Find a safe place and a loving, trusting friend. Take your truth out and share it. Kick it around a bit, on *your* terms. The results will be remarkable.

One sometimes surprising and nearly inevitable side effect of this type of self-disclosure, when done in a safe relationship, is intimacy. As you learned in chapter 6, spirituality and connectedness (and, by extension, intimacy) are essential to releasing your cravings. That's why this second quadrant is so essential to dealing with cravings. Remarkably, the very information that you are afraid of sharing because it might push people away is itself the cement that binds friendships and creates the opportunity for true intimacy and connectedness. This is the healthy way that wounds become scars.

You have another set of truths about you that you are not aware of. Everyone has these. Nobody can see everything about themselves, and without the perspective of others (even if they aren't always right—and they aren't), we would certainly be blind. So the things that others know about you that you cannot or do not see in yourself belong in the third quadrant, the "blind" quadrant. These truths are in your blind spot. Finally, there are aspects of yourself that neither you nor those around you have figured out, and these go in quadrant 4, which is called "unknown."

Ever since those two psychologists developed this way of looking at what is known and unknown about ourselves, this technique has been used in nearly every addiction treatment setting. The reasons are simple. First, since we all suffer from cognitive bias (as explained in chapter 3), the Johari window offers a useful way of seeing that there is much about us that we don't see but that others do. Because this is true, we may be able to start getting glimpses of the side that we are currently blind to by simply asking others for their insight/ perspective and genuinely listening. You can't trust everything someone else says about you, but if several people whom you trust make observations about you that are consistent, they are worth paying attention to, *especially if you disagree with them.* In addiction treatment settings, you will often hear this adage:

> If one person says you're a duck, you can safely dismiss him. If another says it, you might want to pay attention. If a third person says you are a duck, better start quacking.

Actually, ducklings don't begin quacking until several weeks after birth. They have to grow up a bit first. Exploring and facing what others know about you, and what you may not know about yourself, is an important part of growing up emotionally, and, as I've noted before, the fundamental problems of life are never really solved— they are outgrown.

Of course, your friends and the people you trust will also have a limited ability to offer you their perspective if you are keeping secret or hidden important facts about yourself. Your reasons for keeping secrets might be very good ones, or they could simply be driven by anxiety and fear. Either way, if you can't tell the people you really trust about these parts of yourself, they won't be able to help you. Perhaps more important, that degree of secrecy can be a source and a symptom of shame that, as I noted earlier, is toxic and partly responsible for driving cravings. I want to emphasize again that this is not a recommendation to tell everyone your darkest secrets. But if there isn't one nonjudgmental, trustworthy person in your life whom you can count on and open up to, maybe it's time to try and form such a relationship. In Twelve Step programs it can be a sponsor, in religions it can be a pastor or other spiritual leader, and for many it's their counselor—or even their hairdresser. Regardless of who it is, you need to have someone in your life you can trust; someone who will tell you the truth as they see it, even if it hurts your feelings; someone who won't shame or judge you, won't criticize or blame you, but will simply offer you their frank, honest appraisal of your situation. When you find such a person (or persons) and feel confident that you can trust them, you've got to tell them the truth about yourself. This truth includes your secrets, the dark spots, the stuff you are perhaps most ashamed of, maybe even the stuff you swore you'd never tell another human being. Religions have emphasized the value of confession, and psychologists, psychoanalysts, therapists, and psychiatrists have often noted that, without the truth, little progress can be achieved. And in Twelve Step groups, a frequently heard adage is "Your secrets keep you sick." In my experience, these observations are very true. The more you can illuminate these hidden aspects of yourself in a safe, trusting relationship, the easier it will be for you to surrender and step off the craving cycle.

The journey of becoming free from cravings requires change and growth. Certain aspects of yourself you cannot know right now, and your friends and trusted loved ones can't see them either. These are elements of yourself that may become uncovered over time, as you grow and learn more about who you are. That's what the fourth quadrant of the Johari window, the "unknown" quadrant, is all about. The Johari window offers an invitation to discover, explore, change, and ultimately grow. In my experience working with addicts, as you do you will learn things about yourself that you couldn't imagine when you began. You will grow emotionally and react to life in a more mature and fulfilling manner.

Perhaps the most important role that the Johari window can play in combating the naïve perception of immunity is to awaken you to the idea that you really may not know enough about yourself and your cravings to prevent you from acting out on them. I'm not trying to be pessimistic or crush hope, but experience confirms that it's often when you think you've got it all figured out that you are most vulnerable and most at risk. If you can broaden your perspective enough to see that you might need help from others, then you can begin to develop some resiliency against being tricked yet again by your cravings.

The Risks That Accompany Success

It's worth mentioning that you're actually most at risk of the naïve perception of immunity when things are going well. For example, consider the alcoholic who has been sober for three months and is about to relapse by taking her first drink in ninety days. At the moment, things are going great. She has never felt better. She's so glad she's finally licked the alcohol problem. She's been rehired at her job, and her marriage and family life have improved as well. She is even getting back on the beam financially. If you were to do a physical exam on her, you'd find she is in great shape. Her blood pressure is finally normal, and if you took a breathalyzer reading at that moment, it would read 0.000, just as it has every day for the last ninety days. She is sober, and by all outward appearances, she is doing great.

However, if you could read her mind, you would find that it tells a different story. In her mind are a variety of thoughts placing her at extreme risk of taking that first drink (and the ones that inevitably follow) and ruining her sobriety. For some people the thought might be "I'm finally okay; I've proven I don't *need* alcohol." For others it could be "I don't care—I deserve a drink." Other lies that your brain can generate may involve a desire to celebrate, commiserate, take the edge off, "prove" that you don't really have a drinking problem, or confirm that you had been overreacting to the problem. These types of lies can come in every form you could imagine, and then some. Often they occur after a period of success or when things are calm. On the other hand, they may occur in response to stress. These thoughts can even be so subtle that you don't notice them. The one thing they have in common is that they serve to convince you to take the first drink (or that first cigarette, or that first piece of cheesecake, or whatever your craving is). And that's the naïve perception of immunity.

One particularly dangerous idea that sometimes develops in people who are about to relapse and give in to their cravings is the sense that if they can just learn enough or acquire enough information, they'll be able to fix their craving problem, or resist their urges, or choose something different than the object of their cravings. Sometimes this comes in the form of believing they can think through, rationalize, or talk their way out of any craving-related thoughts. To be sure, information and knowledge are important. You do need to learn which actions will be helpful in eliminating your cravings and the chance that you will act on them if they do recur. But the idea that facts alone can solve your problem and eliminate the ongoing need to change your behavior is the essence of naïveté and overconfidence. A prominent Ukrainian geneticist named Theodosius Dobzhansky said, "Scientists often have a naive faith that if only they could discover enough facts about a problem, these facts would somehow arrange themselves in a compelling and true solution." In this case, that solution is ongoing action.

So it seems that you are most likely to believe you are immune when things are going well. Does that mean you should be constantly afraid of achievement and never be able to enjoy your successes? Does it mean you can never regain confidence? No, the truth is just the opposite. The secret lies in the difference between confidence and overconfidence.

On the face of it, overconfidence might seem to be the same as confidence, only too much of it. However, confidence and overconfidence are more different than similar. The sense that you no longer need to form healthy habits, that you can simply resist on your own, and that you can revert to old patterns of behavior is overconfidence. The notion that your craving was a phase, a temporary problem, and now you can finally rest is overconfidence. The belief "If I can just acquire enough information about cravings, I'll be okay" is overconfidence. Overconfidence is naïve. It's this very overconfidence that results in the naïve perception of immunity. Overconfidence is extremely dangerous, and everyone is at risk of experiencing it. The most extreme version of overconfidence is hubris. This type of false pride is responsible for much of the relapse or return to compulsive behavior we see when it comes to craving and addictive behaviors.

So what exactly does healthy confidence look like? What are the characteristics of someone who is experiencing true confidence? First of all, it's important to have some real success in dealing with the craved behavior. A few days or weeks of improvement in a behavior usually aren't enough. If it's been two weeks since you last acted out on your craving, there is much to celebrate, and you should be proud and keep up the great work. But that's usually far too short to result in real, healthy confidence.

There is no definitive cutoff for how long a new behavior pattern should last before it leads to healthy confidence, but in my experience it's rarely weeks or a few months. Usually (but not always), it takes many months or years. The key is to develop enough abstinence or success in eliminating the craved behavior to be confident, but to always be vigilant against overconfidence. Another aspect of healthy confidence is that healthy behaviors and habits no longer feel mostly like chores; rather, they will usually become joyful and something you look forward to. You may find yourself as attracted to the actions that produce success as the success itself. You'll learn more about this in chapter 10, when we'll explore joy, hope, and recovery. But to give you a sense of what to look forward to, you can begin to trust that your confidence is not overconfidence when the actions you took to develop your behavior change and reduce your cravings—the actions that produced these joyous results—are themselves fairly consistently joyful and pleasant. I call it being in the confidence zone.

If going to groups is now a bright spot in your week, something you look forward to instead of it being a chore, then you may be in the confidence zone. If reaching out and asking for help no longer feels like a burden, but something you enjoy doing, you may be in the confidence zone. If spiritually focused behaviors, as I've described them in chapter 6, are actions that you want to do more of rather than less of, then you may be in the confidence zone. And because sometimes you may want to take these actions more than at other times, it really is a zone. It's perfectly normal to hover between wanting to do these actions and not feeling like it. Gaining freedom from cravings is a process. But if you want to take constructive actions more often than not, you're in the zone. That's because confidence is *not* a change in what you do or what you believe you are capable of doing. True confidence is a change in what you *want* to do, and what's most remarkable about it is that it occurs as the result of the kinds of actions described in this book. It's a change in your attitude, not toward the object of your cravings, but toward the very behaviors that help resolve the cravings, in the parlance of AA members "one day at a time."

In Twelve Step meetings, newcomers often ask, "How long do I need to go to these meetings?" One answer that old-timers (those who have achieved substantial success and recovery—usually years or even decades of sobriety) will often give them is "Go until you want to go, and then go some more." The essence of that recommendation is the change in attitude we have been discussing. That's the secret. The real solution to the sense that you are immune, the perception that often comes on strongly when you are doing well, is simply this: *the actions you take to produce recovery will themselves be as desirable to you as the thing you originally craved.* I'm aware that this may sound completely crazy or impossible to you right now. The experience of thousands of recovering people confirms that finding release from cravings is a fundamental change in what you want, which is produced by what you do—*not* the other way around. And that's what is so amazing about gaining freedom from cravings: the process sustains and fuels itself. One simple example of this is when people improve their fitness and health through exercise. At first it's a chore, but gradually it becomes an activity they do because they enjoy it, not because they have to. The action is more of a driver than the result, yet the result continues. Actions change desires, healing produces more healing, and connectedness and spirituality are both the drivers and the results of recovery. You will learn much more about this powerful cycle in chapter 10.

* * *

In this book you have read many examples of people who suffered from cravings and gave in to them despite their best attempts to "be good." The paradox is that when they are occurring, cravings feel like they will last forever; when they go away, it feels like they will never return. Time and again people succumb to this vicious cycle, this roller coaster, without ever being able to step off. In this chapter, you've learned about a particularly devastating aspect of this cycle: that people who suffer from cravings often believe they are immune because they have discovered precisely what they need to stop acting out on their craving. It's that very belief that renders them most vulnerable. By taking steps to become aware of your blind spots, and not simply trusting your own gut when it comes to cravings, you can begin the process of stepping off that self-destructive roller coaster.

. . .

9

Apparently Irrelevant Decisions (AIDs)
How Simple Actions Can Reduce Cravings

*"If you do not change direction, you may end up
where you are heading."*

— LAO TZU

What you believe affects what you want. Even more so, what you do affects what you want. In chapter 3 we reviewed that, in certain cases—and contrary to popular belief—when what you want is out of reach, you actually want it *less*. In this chapter, we'll be exploring how simple actions you take, many of which seem irrelevant, can actually affect your cravings. Many of the recommendations I make will even seem counterintuitive, but they are backed by scientific evidence. Remember that your intuitive responses while in the throes of your cravings may actually be partially responsible for fueling your cravings, so it will sometimes be necessary to do things that run counter to your common sense if you are to successfully lick your cravings.

Apparently Irrelevant Decisions
The father of craving research, the late Dr. Alan Marlatt, used the term "apparently irrelevant decisions" (which he called AIDs) to describe the actions that people with addiction sometimes take that don't seem to them to be related to their cravings but that actually lead to their relapse. The technical name for this is "covert

antecedents." The original example that Marlatt used was an alcoholic who was sober, but who purchased a bottle of alcohol "in case guests dropped by." Marlatt used apparently irrelevant decisions to describe the actions that lead to relapse, but what I'm proposing takes it several steps further. It turns out that many of the actions you can use to *reduce* your cravings will also be apparently irrelevant. Let's look at some of them.

Removing access to the object of craving is, of course, critical, especially early on in your process. If you hadn't read this book, you might have drawn the conclusion that removing access to the object of craving would usually make you want it more. Scientific evidence, however, suggests otherwise.

Although there are exceptions, if you are trying to lose weight, it's probably a bad idea to get a job at Krispy Kreme. If you are trying to stop drinking, being a bartender is probably not the best option. And if you are trying to quit gambling, you may want to find a job far from the Vegas strip. Creating the awareness that the self-destructive behavior is truly off limits can be very helpful in managing cravings. In fact, in what is now considered to be a classic study by Dr. Roger Meyer, only 50 percent of alcoholics craved alcohol when exposed to the sight, smell, or even touch of their favorite beverage if they *knew that they would not be able to drink it.* The mere fact that the alcohol was completely off limits reduced the craving.[107] Behavioral economic research shows similar effects with alcohol price escalation, suggesting that the mere difficulty of obtaining the object of the craving can also reduce cravings. Of course, there are situations where removing access increases desire, but by and large it's likelier that "out of sight, out of mind" will be effective.

In another study of flight attendants who were nicotine dependent, their cravings were measured during two-leg short flights versus long flights. The short flights were about half as long as the long flights. The flight attendants' cravings for cigarettes increased as they approached landing in the short and long flights, but not halfway through the long flights, suggesting that time of abstinence alone doesn't predict craving as well as the sense that they were about to land. In that study, the effect of anticipating the post-landing cigarette was really quite significant.[108] From that study, and several others, we can conclude that context is extremely important and that planning, anticipating, and creating access to the object of your cravings can really ramp up cravings.

What you believe about your cravings can also predict whether you will act on them. In 2010, Australian researcher Nicole Lee and her colleagues assessed 214 methamphetamine users, focusing specifically on what they believed about their cravings. I recently asked Lee about her research, and she explained that when using a questionnaire called the Craving Beliefs Questionnaire, she found a relationship between the addicts' beliefs about their cravings and the probability of relapse.[109] This suggests that addicts who believe that cravings themselves have a detrimental effect on them or their risk of relapse are more likely to return to drug use. In my experience, a simple awareness that cravings are *serious but definitely manageable* helps people commit to other strategies that ensure abstinence. It's my sincere hope that you, too, can gain such awareness, as that very belief (which has the added advantage of being true) may help you stay away from the object of your craving.

Again, although it may seem to you that staying away from what you crave will increase your craving, research suggests just the opposite: the longer you can maintain abstinence, no matter how you do it, the less you crave. A recent study of 865 methamphetamine addicts followed over a four-month period of abstinence showed a clear, dramatic reduction in cravings over time.[110]

Of course, abstinence alone does not produce recovery; this explains why so many people with addiction released from long prison sentences return to drug use before they even arrive home. One study of former smokers who had been abstinent up to ten years showed ongoing cravings in about 10 percent of them, even many years later.[111] People who continued to crave tended to have a more severe history of nicotine dependence and to have more mental health problems. Abstinence is very helpful but hardly enough. Other research has suggested that non-cue-induced cravings do diminish over time, but cue-induced cravings are slower to diminish. (That cigarette display in the gas station tends to "speak" to recovering nicotine addicts for quite a while.)[112] This is why I always emphasize that if you are tempted to test yourself by being exposed to a cue or trigger, you should reconsider. Life contains enough tests—you don't need to add your own.

No one solution will work for all cravings; however, many actions that reduce cravings can be deceptively simple. It can really seem like there is no way that these could work, and yet they do. For example, simply imagining your favorite activity as vividly as you can, can dramatically reduce cravings for food and cigarettes.[113] Several recent studies have shown that the scent of peppermint can reduce cravings for food and nicotine. Mindfulness exercises have also been shown to reduce cravings and substance use.[114] Long-established research shows that stress induces cravings (and this is only partly related to hormonal effects), so any strategies that reduce stress are also very helpful.

I strongly believe that many people with addiction will not be able to completely suppress cravings through cognitive (that is, thinking) methods. Nevertheless, these techniques can be extremely helpful, and they seem to affect the same regions of the brain that are involved in reward that you learned about in chapter 2. In a recent study, people with cocaine cravings attempted to suppress their cravings using cognitive therapy strategies, which functional imaging studies showed reduced the activity in their nucleus accumbens and orbitoprefrontal cortex.[115] That's a fancy way of saying that just using thinking-based methods to suppress cravings affects the parts of the brain involved in craving and reward.

If you don't exercise, you are probably sick of hearing experts extol the benefits of exercise. Add me to the list of those experts. Several studies show the beneficial impact of exercise on craving, and my experience confirms that it can really help. Recently, a small study demonstrated that exercise reduced cravings for marijuana, even in people who weren't seeking treatment for marijuana addiction.[116] Another recent small but rigorous placebo-controlled double-blind study showed benefits of one gram of daily oral acetyl-L-carnitine in alcohol cravings and a higher abstinence rate at ninety days.[117] This compound is thought to somehow be involved in the beneficial effects of exercise. (But don't get me wrong—I don't think we are anywhere near exercise in a pill!)

Many decades of treatment experience confirm that the simple act of talking about a craving helps reduce its intensity and duration. Over the years, I have worked with many people who really struggled to talk about their cravings. The result was usually that these secret cravings became longer, more severe, and more likely to lead to acting out or giving in to the craving. A common belief among these people is that talking about a craving won't help or that talking about it might make it worse. This belief is reinforced by the fact that the few times they discussed their cravings, the cravings *may* have gotten worse. However, the worsening may have been related to some other factor that they aren't recalling, or the connection could be muddled by the attribution biases that we discussed in chapter 3. The extreme example of this belief is when alcoholics tell me that they don't want to attend AA meetings because "talking about alcohol makes me want to drink." It is true that AA meetings vary in how much they focus on illness versus recovery, and I always counsel alcoholics to try to find solution-focused meetings. However, for most alcoholics, any meeting is usually better than no meeting (of course, there are exceptions). I also think that if AA meetings make you want to drink, what hope do you have in the real world, filled with bars, friends who drink, alcohol in foods, billboards and television ads, drinking at sporting events and weddings, and so on? For the majority of alcoholics who benefit from the AA method, it's important to push past this perception and keep attending.

It is very important to talk about cravings. But talking about them in the wrong environment can sometimes do more harm than good. One of the worst mistakes that people make is discussing their cravings with someone who is critical, shaming, or judgmental. I've often seen people who struggled with cravings finally agree to talk to someone about it and end up telling someone who responds with disgust, dismissal, or derogatory comments. I don't think this is an accident—there are powerful unconscious forces that may lead you to seek out judgmental people to discuss your cravings, even though (or perhaps *because*) such discussions are likely to lead to further shaming. As we discussed earlier, shame plays a key role in addiction, and a response like that can intensify shame and subsequently cravings. On balance, however, it's a good idea to talk about your cravings, particularly when you can speak to someone who understands or has been there.

The deceptively simple act of saying that you are craving, out loud, to someone who really understands can sometimes make the difference between success and suffering. However, as members of Twelve Step fellowships have noted for decades, sometimes the telephone can weigh a hundred pounds. In other words, in the midst of the craving, it can be very difficult to initiate behaviors such as making a phone call to an understanding friend. This may also be due, in part, to prefrontal cortex effects described in chapter 2.

Thus, the old adage that the time to fix the roof is when it's not raining applies to cravings as well. Establishing a habit of discussing your goals, successes, and struggles on a daily basis (whether or not you are craving) will make it much easier to make the call when the craving hits. Again, the power of the group, as we reviewed in chapter 7, can be leveraged for success in dealing with cravings.

Many members of self-help and mutual-help groups learned this long ago and emphasize the importance of getting phone numbers and regularly connecting with others who struggle. The fear that such discussions will trigger additional cravings (which, by the way, can occur) is outweighed by the overwhelming benefits of this type of interpersonal connection and the extraordinary ability of the group to achieve what the individual often cannot.

Another cognitive distortion that interferes with the simple and successful act of talking about your cravings is the belief that "if I don't think about it, it will go away." This powerful but dangerous belief has resulted in many heartbreaking relapses or a return to the unhealthy behavior, as the sense that what's really needed is to simply forget about the self-destructive behavior crowds out the more rational suggestion that taking simple actions is the best way to prevent and manage cravings.

Actions to Prevent and Manage Cravings

Help Others

The core "rediscovery" made by early AA members was that helping others reduces the desire to drink. These two things may seem unrelated. While helping people is a good thing, of course, what could it possibly have to do with cravings?

We continue to learn about the important role of helping others in reducing cravings, but the simple idea that helping others can help our cravings leads us to the next suggestion of an apparently irrelevant action that can suppress cravings: help someone. A recent study of 195 addicted adolescents found that helping others during treatment was linked to substantially improved substance abuse outcomes.[118] One of the cofounders of Alcoholics Anonymous, Dr. Bob Smith, in his farewell talk before he died, noted that "Our Twelve Steps, when simmered down to the last, resolve themselves into the words 'love' and 'service.'" As we noted in chapter 3, love neutralizes shame, and service to others (in other words, helpfulness) reduces obsession and craving. The fundamental observation that serving others reduces cravings is actually much older than AA, which is why I call it a rediscovery. Lao Tzu wrote, in the *Tao Te Ching*:

> The Master has no possessions.
> The more he does for others,
> the happier he is.
> The more he gives to others,
> the wealthier he is.

Each of these suggestions can make a difference in your cravings, but don't fall prey to the idea that any one of them will solve your problem. The exclusive reliance on helpfulness to others to manage cravings has resulted in many avoidable relapses. I have seen many recovering alcoholics who work as counselors, treatment center directors, and medical directors of addiction rehabs go through relapse. Often these people were involved in tireless service to others precisely when the relapse occurred. They were then very surprised that service and helpfulness to others did not stave off their cravings and prevent relapse.

In many of these cases, these were active participants in recovery programs who stopped attending meetings or participating in recovery-related activities outside of their workplace. They erroneously concluded that the service they did at work would be sufficient for them to maintain sobriety. In interviewing dozens of such individuals, I have learned that they often began to see themselves as fundamentally different from the people they were helping. The treatment principle of therapeutic distance (the importance of maintaining social boundaries with the people we help) reinforced that. Often these people also started feeling uncomfortable at recovery meetings that their own patients were also attending. As a result, they simply stopped going, and later relapsed. It turns out that this is so common that most sensible employers of recovering counselors consider this line of work to be an occupational hazard, and AA has even published guidelines suggesting that members maintain their own personal AA lives outside of their work environment.[119]

The role of service within recovering communities cannot be overemphasized. Long-standing sober members of these communities have noted the importance of making coffee, setting up chairs, leading meetings, cleaning up afterward, and other types of helpfulness as key to their ongoing success.

For another helpful action to reduce cravings, consider this adage: "If you want self-esteem, take 'esteemable' actions." It's particularly true for people who suffer from cravings. As shame is endemic to addicts, addressing it is crucial to reduce ongoing cravings and relapse. This may be, in part, why taking and sharing one's "moral inventory" and making amends are so essential to Twelve Step recovery (Steps 4, 5, 8, and 9 of the Twelve Step program). The guilt, shame, and resentment from years of self-destructive behavior emerge in the form of obsession and craving, and serve to disrupt success in recovering from addictions. (By the way, *self-destructive behavior* is in some ways a terrible term, as it downplays the hurtful nature of these behaviors toward others.)

In general, attempts to explain the role that the ingredients of Twelve Step programs play in establishing and maintaining abstinence are usually misguided, incomplete, or grossly oversimplified. This is reflected in the partially sarcastic response that some members give to the question "How does it work?" "It works just fine." Nevertheless, there are core features of Twelve Step programs that can, in my experience, be extracted for the benefit of others who suffer from various cravings.

Avoid Dangerous Situations

Another useful suggestion for dealing with cravings is to *avoid dangerous situations*. The hardest part about this suggestion is that you may not know what's dangerous. If you trust your gut, situations that feel safe may simply feel that way because they are familiar but are, in fact, very risky. You may also fall prey to a trick your mind plays on you that convinces you that you need to "test" your recovery to determine if you can handle these situations. Those tests don't often go well. This is one of the reasons that so many recovery programs emphasize sharing with others and obtaining an accountability partner to run your ideas and plans by. To really know what's unsafe, you'll need to autopsy your relapses: What was happening before you gave in? What was your state of mind? And what other environmental factors were at play?

I always recommend that my patients ask themselves, "Am I ASPHALT (anxious, scared, preoccupied, hungry, angry, lonely, or tired)?" Were you having negative thoughts about yourself? Or perhaps just the opposite: were you wanting to celebrate something? All of the circumstances leading up to your acting out on the craving need to be inventoried, and for that you'll need help, someone nonjudgmental but compassionate enough to genuinely listen and courageous enough to tell you the truth.

Finding the right person can be a challenge for some people. They may have taught themselves over the years that being vulnerable is dangerous, having impulsively placed themselves in vulnerable positions and thus repeatedly had their trust violated. If you are someone who feels like people often betray you and that "nobody can be trusted," consider seeking professional help in finding the right person to open up to.

Develop Healthy Habits and Routines

Yet another helpful suggestion for managing cravings is to form new habits and routines. As you've seen throughout this book, old habits can often very subtly lead to acting out on cravings and can increase the chance of experiencing cravings. In general, habits aren't forgotten, but replaced. Think of habits as recordings on magnetic tape. The only way to remove them is to write over them. Another way of thinking of habits is as grooves. To really solidify them, they have to be repeated. That process etches them in. If you decide that a particular action is helpful to your efforts to gain freedom from cravings, do it on a set schedule. Go to the same meetings each week, call your support person at the same time every week, and so on. This will make you more resilient to the effects of stress and impulsivity. Although this type of routine may seem unnecessary or unrelated to your cravings, do it anyway. When times get tough, your car will do a better job of steering itself away from a danger zone if you have new habits in place.

Many of the suggestions I've already made for helping with your cravings may sound apparently irrelevant. Connecting to others in a group, being accountable, and being helpful to others may not intuitively seem related to freedom from cravings, but as we showed earlier, they definitely are.

Find a Sense of Purpose

Here is another suggestion that can really make a difference in reducing cravings and the risk of acting out on them: develop a sense of purpose. Having a purpose, a mission statement, or a clear goal can motivate you, ground you, and give you a sense of focus that can help you deal with cravings and stay connected to your recovery program. Once again, we can turn to AA and other Twelve Step groups for examples. AA states that its primary purpose is for its members to stay sober and help other alcoholics achieve sobriety. Its textbook *Alcoholics Anonymous* states, "Our real purpose is to fit ourselves to be of maximum service to God and the people about us."[120] The purpose of Celebrate Recovery (a Christian-based recovery program) is to "fellowship and celebrate God's healing power in our lives." Similarly, secular organizations focused on recovery have purpose statements. If you can develop a sense of purpose, it will certainly help you as you work toward freedom from cravings.

Meet Your Needs in a Healthy Way

Throughout this book I've emphasized that what seems unrelated to cravings can often be exactly what you need to look at or focus on. Your cravings thrive, in part, because your brain has learned to selectively ignore the things that are driving them. Many of the actions you need to take in order to get well are "apparently irrelevant." There is another way of looking at this important phenomenon that may be very helpful as you develop your own plan to reduce or eliminate your cravings, and it's based on the following principle: if you don't meet your needs in a healthy way, you *will* meet them artificially. That usually means that you will crave self-destructive ways of meeting your needs. In fact, most of the suggestions I've been giving you to address your cravings are designed to meet these very needs in a new, healthier way.

Let's take a closer look at what that means. If you think of all the things you need to live a happy, fulfilling, and joyous life, you can generally divide them into twenty categories.

	PHYSICAL	EMOTIONAL	MENTAL	SPIRITUAL
Security	Physical security	Emotional security	Mental security	Spiritual security
Identity	Physical identity	Emotional identity	Mental identity	Spiritual identity
Intimacy	Physical intimacy	Emotional intimacy	Mental intimacy	Spiritual intimacy
Creativity	Physical creativity	Emotional creativity	Mental creativity	Spiritual creativity
Adventure	Physical adventure	Emotional adventure	Mental adventure	Spiritual adventure

When you look at this table, you might think, "Those sound interesting, but do I really *need* all of those things? I thought I only needed food, shelter, clothing, water, and love. Do I need emotional creativity or mental adventure? Do I really need physical adventure and spiritual identity?" You shouldn't be surprised that you are asking yourself those questions. Chances are pretty good that if you don't think you need those things, then you probably are not meeting those needs, and that could be driving your cravings, even if the connection is apparently irrelevant to you.

What do these categories actually represent? Let's look at some examples. It turns out that you do need mental intimacy. You need to connect with other people around what you think and how you think. If you have ideas in life (about how to take care of yourself, how to be helpful, or what might make life a little more fun, for example), then you need to share those with others. If you keep your ideas to yourself (which does happen sometimes, especially when a person believes that their thoughts are worthless or that nobody would care to hear them), then your fundamental need for mental intimacy is not being met.

Similarly, you need to experience emotional adventure. If you just emotionally squeak by in life, never allowing yourself to take emotional risks and experience the full range of emotions, suppressing them or always trying to rigidly control how you feel, you will not meet your fundamental need for emotional adventure.

In just the same way, you can examine each of these basic needs. I can assure you that if you ignore any one of these areas (and most people ignore *most* of them), then you will run into serious problems that will seem to be entirely unrelated to that particular need category. This is because of the fundamental axiom that if you don't meet your needs in a healthy way, you *will* meet them in an artificial way. It could be a late-night sugar binge, a gambling spree, another cigarette, or any other unhealthy craving. We've all heard of "emotional eating." In my experience, this type of eating is rarely simply "emotional." Rather, it's a result of not meeting several of your fundamental needs.

If you ask yourself how well you are currently meeting each of these twenty needs (rate each one on a scale of 1–5, with 5 being extremely well and 1 being not at all), you'll get a sense of what areas to focus on first. Take the areas where you scored less than 3 and ask yourself what you are doing to meet those basic needs and what you could do in order to meet them. I've worked with people who have identified specific actions they could take to address these unmet needs. For one man it was taking drawing classes, as he was always afraid of drawing (he had rated himself a 2 on physical creativity). A woman I worked with decided to try skydiving because of her low self-rating on physical adventure. For another young man it was working up the courage to finally ask someone out on a date (emotional intimacy), and for yet another it was signing up to volunteer with the Big Brother program. These are the actions that these individuals decided to take, and they won't necessarily be right for your program. But by making a focused, concerted effort to work on their basic needs, they were able to take care of themselves at an extremely high level. Because they were taking care of their needs in a healthy way, their brains and bodies no longer needed to try to meet those needs in an artificial way (like binge eating, for example). Their shame dissolved, and their acting out on their cravings diminished or completely disappeared. Most of the recommendations I've made in this book are designed to help you meet many of these needs. For example, Twelve Step meeting attendance and Twelve Step program participation can help you meet a large number of these needs, although recovery is *not* one size fits all.

The amazing thing about these solutions to cravings is that they can seem entirely unrelated to the problem if you don't grasp the underlying processes. Fortunately, you don't actually need to understand these processes for the solutions to work; you just need to take the actions. But if you want to make sense of them, it helps to know the *why* behind them. When something is a need, it's not optional. Your needs will be satisfied. If you don't meet your needs in a way that is helpful to you, they will be met in a way that is not helpful to you. They will not, however, be ignored. Through my experience helping people with cravings, I've discovered the ridiculously simple and obvious truth that your needs really are necessary. If you do not achieve emotional intimacy in a healthy way, for example, your brain will demand that it be satisfied in an artificial way (which could be a pint of Ben and Jerry's, another cigarette, or a trip to the slot machines). You might be able to put it off for a while, but in the end you won't really have a choice. The need will be satisfied one way or another. Why not seek relief by identifying your needs and meeting them in a productive, satisfying, and healthy way?

. . .

10

Joy, Hope, and Recovery

"You were born with wings—Why prefer to crawl through life?"

— JALAL AD-DIN RUMI

By now you've learned that a combination of nature (genetics) and nurture (environment) are responsible for cravings, and changes in your brain fuel addictive behaviors. You've learned that your brain tricks you into believing things that aren't true—things about yourself, about your cravings, and about what it takes for you to be satisfied. You've learned that there is no shortage of ways that your brain lies to you to undermine your success in releasing your cravings.

But you've also learned that there are specific actions you can take to change your brain in ways that can bring relief from cravings and get you started on a path to experience a sense of joy and hope that is nothing short of extraordinary. Yes, many of these specific actions may seem unnecessary or even counterintuitive, but it's this very sense that the actions won't work, aren't necessary, or don't make sense that has been blocking you from making the changes you need to achieve freedom from self-destructive cravings.

We've all met dry drunks or people who are "white knuckling" (using the sheer force of will to resist cravings). These folks are often bitter and resentful, or contemptuous and angry. In many such cases, the friends and loved ones of these people often liked them better when they were not resisting their cravings! That's not recovery and freedom. For this process to be worth it, eliminating or resisting cravings is not enough. The recovery process cannot simply be about stopping something. Most people who have achieved successful, long-term, contented release from cravings and addictive behaviors report that recovery is about 5 percent what you stop doing and 95 percent what you start doing.

As mentioned earlier in this book, some people achieve recovery through religion, others through a transformative experience, and still others through group aid such as Twelve Step programs or SMART recovery. Sadly, much energy has been wasted as members of these various organizations bicker with each other about which works best, and this leaves the newcomer perplexed about which camp to believe, as everywhere he goes one group's members seem to be debunking another's. A recent examination by my colleague Mark Willenbring, M.D., one of the world's foremost authorities on alcoholism, concluded that over 20 million Americans are in recovery from addiction to alcohol and drugs. I can tell you this much: they didn't all do it the same way.

I have seen people who suffer from cravings for alcohol, drugs, tobacco, gambling, compulsive eating, compulsive exercise, and even self-destructive sex patterns achieve joyful, contented recoveries in many different ways. If you are a hammer, everything looks like a nail. So members of the various self-help and mutual-aid organizations often seem to privately believe that theirs is the only reasonable approach, even if they publicly proclaim that they don't own the only solution.

The key to a joyful, hope-filled, and contented life free of cravings and addiction is to look past the noise and find the approach that works for you. That does *not* necessarily mean the path that feels right. Often the method that feels most comfortable is not challenging you enough on the areas that really need to change. So I always advise my patients to find what works, not necessarily what's comfortable, especially at first, when the discomfort of change is actually most needed. And that means finding people who have been successful, whom you can trust, and then sticking close to them. It also means laying the groundwork to render yourself truly open to feedback from others whom you trust.

A common saying in AA is that if you wrote down everything you expected from recovery when newly sober, sealed it in an envelope, and then opened it years later, you would find that you had sold yourself short. Over and over again I hear from people who have achieved long-term freedom from their addictive behavior that the life they've obtained as a result of allowing themselves to be transformed and helping others is so much better than they ever could have imagined. I've heard this so many times, in fact, that it seems to be the rule, and anything less is the exception.

In most cases, what seems to limit us is ourselves—our attitudes about how things *should* be, a sense that perhaps we don't deserve better, or a profound underestimation of what we are capable of achieving. This feels true, and yet the real truth is that this underestimation is not and cannot be authentic, because our true selves are far more than we could ever imagine.

Earlier we explored how addictive cravings are shame-based phenomena. Shame, the profound sense that "I am broken" or that "I am worthless," is a devastating force. It eagerly consumes joy, peace, and contentment and renders a person worse than sick—it renders them unable to believe that things could be any other way. In other words, shame destroys hope.

As I've witnessed people's lives be destroyed by shame and then rebuilt by recovery, one thing has been consistently clear: the process of recovering from shame is profoundly courageous. For some people, simply telling themselves that the shame is based on a lie is enough. Affirmations, for example, are one way that many have achieved some relief from the black hole of shame. But for most people who suffer from the shame-craving-shame cycle, self-talk, although helpful, will not be enough.

Shame destroys joy; shame destroys hope; shame destroys peace. Shame destroys connectedness and fosters isolation and loneliness. There is, however, one force that seems to consistently neutralize shame time and again.

What then, destroys shame? The answer is deceptively simple and perhaps counterintuitive. It's love. Love is the force that allows shame sufferers to outgrow shame and transform. Love restores hope and creates the sense of peace and contentment that allows for long-term, happy recovery. What exactly does that look like?

Am I suggesting a return to 1960s free-love, commune-style living where organization and structure are to be vilified and hippie culture worshipped? Don't tie-dye your business suits just yet.

Altruism

Most major movements that have helped people achieve relief from cravings emphasize helpfulness to others and a sense of altruism. Even groups that emphasize the role of self-directedness and self-will in eliminating compulsive and addictive behaviors are primarily driven by people who genuinely enjoy helping others. The sense that we are self-sufficient really isn't true. The love of one's fellow human being and the genuine desire to be of service is core to recovery, central to eliminating cravings, and critical to neutralizing shame. Although most attempts to define spirituality seem to reveal only *our own* limitations rather than telling us anything about what spirituality is, for many who have successfully recovered, another word for spirituality is really *connectedness*.

I've met many people who struggle with addictive behaviors who have told me that they felt alone even when in a roomful of friends. The isolation that cravings and addiction create may sometimes outwardly appear to be a physical isolation, but at its core it's a spiritual and emotional isolation. The old joke that "intimacy is really 'into-me-see'" turns out to be true. Allowing yourself to be seen—eliminating dark, toxic secrets, like cleaning out a wound—is essential to the processes of intimacy, connectedness, and, ultimately, recovery. In recovery talk, recovering addicts describe themselves as "clean." This sense of being clean derives, in part, from losing the toxicity of shameful secrets. This level of closeness to trusted friends, initially terrifying to those who suffer from addiction, becomes not only acceptable but highly desirable.

Recovery, however, usually takes people well beyond connection and toward compassion. For many, the joy of recovery includes a "burning desire" to share what they have gained from personal transformation with others who are still struggling. Earlier we saw how altruism and helpfulness promote reduction in cravings and addictive behaviors. Here, in recovery, we see how the capacity to be helpful is not only a cause of recovery, but a *gift* of recovery, as a certain type of peace and joy derives directly from the act of helping others. A genuine sympathy, and even empathy for others, and a deep, personal striving to reduce the suffering of others are natural consequences of recovery-oriented living.

Finding Your Authentic Self

As I think of compassion and sharing, I'm reminded of the story of John Woolman, an eighteenth-century Quaker from New Jersey who recognized, well ahead of his country, that something his peers were doing did not make moral sense to him: slavery. This awareness alone was not, however, enough for Woolman. His beliefs took him to a point where he would not write a bill of sale for a slave, nor would he use or purchase the products of slavery, which was no mean feat in mid-1700s America.

He found himself compelled to engage other Quakers on this issue in a most remarkable way. He didn't proselytize or argue, and he didn't criticize or judge. Instead, John Woolman went from farm to farm, meeting with Quakers on the East Coast for more than two decades. During this process, he simply asked questions, like "What does it mean to be a moral person?" and "What does it mean to have a slave?" Woolman began this gentle and genuine questioning of his peers in the mid-eighteenth century. By 1770, slavery was almost completely eliminated from Quaker homes, a century before the rest of America would catch up.

John Woolman's authenticity, compassion, courage, and joy were not separate, disconnected ideas. Instead, he found that the act of being true to himself led him to a life where compassion, courage, and joy were inseparable and nearly inevitable. He had let go of selfishness enough to be free of worrying about what others thought of him. While others were blocked by greed, self-centeredness, or fear, he was free to do the right thing. When John Woolman died on October 7, 1772, sadly, slavery was still rampant in America. Despite that, those present with him recorded that his last moments were filled with "the happiness, the safety, and the beauty of a life devoted to following the Heavenly Shepherd."

Communities of recovery have appropriated Shakespeare's "To thine own self be true" and completely transformed its meaning in the process. Being true to oneself, that is to say, being authentic, does not just produce recovery but is also a result of recovery. It's truly a gift to be free of the constant need for the approval of others. In the *Tao Te Ching*, Lao Tzu writes

> Fill your bowl to the brim
> and it will spill.
> Keep sharpening your knife
> and it will blunt.
> Chase after money and security
> and your heart will never unclench.
> Care about people's approval
> and you will be their prisoner.

The surprising result of finding your authentic self is not simply the discovery that you are worthy, but that your essence is worthiness and that compassion, connectedness, authenticity, and love are reflections of that worthy core.

Courage

What will it take to get there? Anaïs Nin said that life shrinks or expands in proportion to one's courage. Twelve Step members frequently refer to "the courage to change." Courage is, in fact, the most essential quality of recovery, because without courage, none of the other needed practices are possible. It's impossible to be authentic without courage. Yet most people have tremendous courage without ever realizing it, and this is certainly true for those who have struggled under the burden of addictions. You are generally the last person to notice your own courage, although you may see courage in others. In my work helping those who suffer from addictions and cravings, I've noticed that people are really blind to their own bravery. In fact, the very act of reading this book is courageous. If you hear that statement and think to yourself, "Nobody would consider reading a book to be courageous," notice that thought. The voice that tells you that you are not courageous, that you cannot do this, that you are ordinary, is precisely what blocks you from recognizing and engaging your own courage. It's the inertia of addictive thinking.

Addictions are fueled by stiffness and inertia. Most people who suffer from them are profoundly afraid of change. They don't want to change their environment, their routines, their habits, or their way of looking at the world. Of course, they want to change the misery, the loneliness, the pain, and the shame, but just can't seem to do that or to do it consistently. The irony is that as much as people who suffer from cravings dislike change, their behaviors and their disease constantly produce precisely the type of changes in their lives that hurt the most. Their rigidity actually fuels self-destructive behavior. For the food addict it might be weight gain, and for the gambling addict, bankruptcy. But one way or another, resisting flexibility and sticking to routine produce changes that are far worse that the ones they were trying to avoid.

Recovery requires flexibility. People in recovery adapt. They are open to new ways of doing things, and as a result become open to new ways of looking at things and, ultimately, new ways of experiencing life. They recognize that context matters, and they are open-minded and willing to challenge themselves. They structure their lives so that they cannot rest on their laurels. They resist the idea that they've figured it out; rather, they are constantly seeking to learn more about themselves and about others. Their experience is like walking up a down escalator. If they stop walking, they will move backward. Many people in recovery describe recovery as a process, a journey, not something that is ever complete, but rather something that involves seeing the new in everything, even in what may be familiar and what may seem ordinary.

The nineteenth-century American poet Walt Whitman wrote in "Song of Myself," "Do I contradict myself? / Very well then I contradict myself, / (I am large, I contain multitudes.)" People healing from craving-related self-destructive behavior can hold opposite ideas without being torn apart. They can say, "I did something I didn't want to do, but that doesn't make me a bad person." They recognize that things are far more amazing and complex than they could ever seem, and yet they are open to seeing the simplicity of things as well. They are aware of the infinite in themselves and their relationships, and in particular recognize that every day offers opportunities to see and experience life in a new, richer way, even if that new experience contradicts what they surely knew to be true yesterday.

I've emphasized connectedness as essential to spirituality. What does it take to connect? Take a moment and reflect on someone you met as an adult but are very close to. Someone you trust and with whom you feel connected. Now ask yourself, what brought you together? Did you say to yourself, "I want to be friends with her because she never makes mistakes?" Of course not. In most cases, we connect around our warts, our imperfections, and our woundedness. Perhaps a common adversity, a shared struggle, or just a tough moment? The truth is, people connect around their brokenness, around their imperfection. Denying our suffering and our pain is not simply inauthentic; it's tragic. The tragedy is that this denial prevents us from accessing the very joy we thought we could attain by ignoring our own wounds. Ernie Kurtz, author of *The Spirituality of Imperfection: Storytelling and the Search for Meaning*, wrote:

> A spirituality of imperfection suggests that spirituality's first step involves facing self squarely, seeing one's self as one is: mixed-up, paradoxical, incomplete, and imperfect. Flawedness is the first fact about human beings. And paradoxically, in that imperfect foundation we find not despair but joy. For it is only within the reality of our imperfection that we can find the peace and serenity we crave.[121]

Allowing your imperfections, then embracing them, and ultimately celebrating them, is an important part of the joy of recovery. These are not new ideas; 2,500 years ago, Lao Tzu said, "If you want to become whole, let yourself be partial. If you want to become straight, let yourself be crooked." Letting go of the need to be perfect and to be right results in a freedom that is otherwise impossible.

Letting Go

So the process of recovery is a process of letting go. A common expression in Twelve Step recovery circles is "Let go and let God." Letting go is not intuitive or obvious; our natural tendency is often to hang on to things that are impeding our growth. I'm reminded of a story, two stories really, that are nearly identical, although they occurred forty-five years apart. The first is the story of a wildfire that occurred in Mann Gulch, Montana, in 1949. The second, nearly identical story is of a wildfire in South Canyon, Colorado. In 1949, thirteen firefighters lost their lives, and in 1994, another fourteen died. In both cases, scientific analysis revealed that these men and women lost their lives because when the fires intensified, and they needed to retreat, *they refused to drop their tools.* They refused to let go. In fact, since 1994, several more firefighters have died for the same reason. There are similar stories among fighter pilots, and this principle has even been used to explain underperformance in everything from athletics to business.

One of my mentors, Dr. Lynn Isabella, Associate Professor of Business Administration at the University of Virginia, pointed out ten reasons why these firefighters did not drop their tools. I won't review all the reasons here, but a few are worth mentioning. First, the firefighters were able to maintain a sense of control by hanging on to the tools. Earlier in this book we learned about cognitive bias and how maintaining a sense of control is so important that people will sometimes destroy themselves just to maintain that feeling.

Second, the firefighters had no skill at a replacement activity. "If I drop my tools, if I let go, what will I do instead?" The things that hold people back are often the only things that feel familiar. People may hang on to self-destructive behaviors because they know and have practiced no other way. Third, for many of the firefighters, a core belief was "we are our tools." People who are early in the recovery process often describe a fear of change because they will lose themselves. They may fear that they *are* their self-destructive behaviors. This is, as I noted above, a distorted belief, because we are so much more than we could ever imagine. Other reasons that these brave men and women didn't let go of their tools included not trusting the messenger that advised them to do it and not wanting to admit failure.

However, the one reason that really stands out is that the firefighters believed that the small changes associated with dropping their tools seemed too trivial to really make a difference. In the 1949 incident, it was calculated that dropping their tools would have enabled them to move 8 inches per second faster. Seems trivial, right? In the end they made it 260 feet. Sadly, safety was at 263 feet.

The same phenomenon happens over and again in people struggling to gain freedom from cravings. On countless occasions people have told me, "That won't make a difference—it's a minor thing." "Do I really need to call someone every day?" "Do I really need to tell someone *all* my secrets?" Many people who struggle with cravings refuse to let go of the things holding them back, only to stop three feet short of safety. In AA parlance, they "quit ten minutes before the miracle."

Don't underestimate the power of letting go. On your new journey of recovery, your practices can help you let go of the need to be right, the need to control, the need to please others. You can let go of the need to always have all the answers. Earlier in this book we learned about the power of habits and the way that these are etched deeper and deeper like grooves. Letting go can help you produce new habits, actions that can support your ongoing growth and recovery from the toxicity that acting out on cravings has produced in your life.

* * *

My experience working with thousands of men and women is that what stands between you and freedom from cravings is mostly related to what you think, but that to change what you think you must change what you do. Recovery is a lifelong journey that involves doing just that.

Best wishes as you progress along your path. If you discover something that might be helpful to others, I'd love to hear from you.

• • •

Finding Help for Alcoholism or Drug Addiction

Are you worried about your drinking or drug use? Is your drinking or drug use negatively affecting other areas of your life? Have you made a decision to stop drinking or using drugs but don't know how to stop? The following list contains resources that can help you.

- Find meetings and information about Alcoholics Anonymous (AA) or Narcotics Anonymous (NA) by going to AA.org or NA.org. Click on the meeting finder to locate a meeting near you. Open meetings are open to everyone. Closed meetings are limited to persons who have a desire to stop drinking or using. You decide which meetings are right for you.

- Family members and loved ones of alcoholics and addicts can attend Al-Anon or Nar-Anon meetings, which can be found at al-anon.org and nar-anon.org.

- Teenagers who have relatives with alcoholism or another addiction can benefit from Alateen. See www.alateen.org for more information.

- Alcoholics and addicts who are interested in Christian-based programs may be interested in Celebrate Recovery. Find out more at www.celebraterecovery.com.

- To learn more about addiction to alcohol and other drugs, including alcohol's affect on your health, underage drinking, fetal alcohol exposure, and other topics, see the brochures, fact sheets, videos, and other educational materials from the National Institute on Alcohol Abuse and Alcoholism (NIAAA) at www.niaaa.nih.gov/publications or the National Institute on Drug Abuse (NIDA) at www.drugabuse.gov. These publications are generally of a very high quality, evidence-based, and informative.

- For those interested in receiving treatment for alcohol or drug abuse, the Substance Abuse and Mental Health Services Administration (SAMHSA) provides an online treatment locator. The locator can be found at http://findtreatment .samhsa.gov.

The Alcohol Use Disorders Identification Test (AUDIT)

The AUDIT screening tool is a short questionnaire created by the World Health Organization that you can take yourself, or for a loved one, to determine whether there's a potential for hazardous drinking, or a need for counseling and/or treatment. You can find the test online at www.integration.samhsa.gov/AUDIT_screener_for_alcohol.pdf.

- A score of 8 or more suggests hazardous or problematic drinking.
- A score of 15 to 19 suggests benefit from brief counseling and support.
- In general, scores of 20 or greater suggest that treatment should be sought.

About My Drinking

Another great resource is www.AboutMyDrinking.org, which is a free, online screening tool offered by Hazelden. The screening tool allows you to see how your alcohol or drug use compares to what's considered healthy use. The site can also connect you with resources, products, and services to help you reduce or stop your drinking or drug use altogether, as well as treatment and recovery services.

. . .

Tips for Specific Cravings

The following section contains tips and information for dealing with specific cravings, including smoking, alcohol, narcotic pain pills (for people with chronic pain), sugar, chocolate, gambling, and the Internet. Try a few of the suggestions to get started and keep trying until you land on one or two that work for you. Some of these techniques will take time to become a part of your routine, so stick with them. You may also find these suggestions lead you to create your own healthy ways of coping with cravings.

Smoking

Trying to quit smoking? The following list contains proactive measures you can take to prevent or lessen your cravings for cigarettes when you are trying to quit.

- **Set a quit date.** Note: there is no time like the present.

- **Tell your friends, colleagues, and loved ones what your quit date is.** Although you may be embarrassed about what they'll say if you relapse, remember that your true friends will support rather than judge you.

- **Remove all smoking paraphernalia from your home, office, car, and anywhere else you go.** This means ashtrays, cigarettes, lighters, matchbooks, even clothing with cigarette logos. Wash your clothes so they don't smell like smoke, and wash your car too. Remember: you are a nonsmoker, and nonsmokers don't smell like smoke.

- **Take medications for smoking cessation.** There are many available, including over-the-counter options like nicotine gums and patches, and prescription options like Zyban and Chantix. These medications are not without risk, so be sure to talk to your physician about them. Remember, however, that quitting success rates are dramatically higher in people who use these types of aids. And it's *not* cheating!

- **Change your routines.** If you smoke with your coworkers, let them know that you won't be joining them and ask them not to invite you. Don't frequent establishments where smoking is permitted. In the early days and weeks of quitting, try not to be alone too much. If the person you are with can support your abstinence, that's great too.

- **Identify an accountability partner.** Preferably this is a trusting, nonjudgmental friend who is willing to provide emotional support during the tough times. It may be someone who has successfully quit. Ask this person if he or she would be willing to check in with you regularly, and if you can call him or her too.

When the craving for a cigarette hits, try one or more of the following to avoid lighting up:

- **Change your environment.** For example, if you're in a bar, go home. If you're in a place or situation that is high-stress, leave.

- **Ask for help.** Call your accountability partner or friend and tell him or her you are craving. Remember: your friend doesn't need to know how to solve the problem for you— the mere act of sharing your craving has been shown to diminish it.

- **Distract yourself and do something else.** Preferably, it would be something productive, like going for a walk, exercising, cleaning the house, or reading. But even a mindless activity like chewing gum or watching TV is better than smoking.

- **Write it down.** If you write down how you are feeling, what you are doing, and what is going on every time you crave a cigarette, you will start to see patterns. Maybe you crave more after sex, after a movie, before dinner, or when you are stressed at work. By identifying high-risk scenarios, you can develop a plan to deal with them the next time they occur.

- **Remind yourself that all cravings end, and that most only last a few minutes.** If it's helpful, carry an index card with these suggestions in your wallet.

- **Grab this book and re-read chapter 10 to give you hope and inspiration.** Or find a different inspirational book. Focusing on the positive will reduce your cravings.

- **Practice mindfulness meditation or other forms of relaxation.** Time and again, stress-reduction techniques have been shown to reduce craving duration and intensity. Find a method that works for you and *practice*!

Alcohol

For those who are in recovery from alcohol addiction, trying to quit for personal or health reasons, or simply attempting to reduce their drinking, the following techniques can help you deal with alcohol cravings and avoid relapse.

- **Leave the situation.** Whether it's a bar, a friend's house, an office party, or even your own home, changing the scene is usually a good idea. When a craving hits, it can be hard to know what exactly triggered it. It's usually best to leave the situation, then try to figure out what sparked the craving later. Sometimes no reason can be found; cravings are common in early sobriety.

- **Call or talk to someone.** Talking about cravings reduces the frequency and intensity of cravings. Discuss them, don't keep them to yourself. Remember, the person you talk to doesn't need to have a solution for the cravings—they just need to lend an understanding ear. Keep many numbers in your cell phone contacts of people who would be willing to talk you through the cravings.

- **Get to a meeting.** If you prefer Twelve Step meetings, get yourself to an AA meeting. If you are receiving support from some other group, go there. Get with like-minded people as soon as possible.

- **Eat. Drink. Rest. Connect.** You've heard me mention anxious-scared-preoccupied-hungry-angry-lonely-tired (ASPHALT) as a recipe for disaster. Counteract these known craving triggers by staying hydrated, staying well-fed, resting, and connecting as much as possible with healthy, supportive people. You can't rely on your body's own signals during a craving, so eat a healthy snack and drink (nonalcoholic) fluids even if you aren't hungry or thirsty.

- **Keep a list of reasons you are quitting in your wallet.** Refer to them often, not just during the cravings.

- **Change your environment.** For example, if you're in a bar, go home. If you're in a place or situation that is high-stress, leave.

- **Distract yourself and do something else.** Preferably, it would be something productive like going for a walk, exercising, cleaning the house, or reading. But even a mindless activity like chewing gum or watching TV is better than taking a drink.

- **Write it down.** If you write down how you are feeling, what you are doing, and what is going on every time you crave a drink, you will start to see patterns. Maybe you crave more after sex, after a movie, before dinner, or when you are stressed at work. By identifying high-risk scenarios, you can develop a plan to deal with them the next time they occur.

- **Remind yourself that all cravings end, and that most only last a few minutes.** If it's helpful, carry an index card with these suggestions in your wallet.

- **Grab this book and re-read chapter 10 to give you hope and inspiration.** Or find a different inspirational book. Focusing on the positive will reduce your cravings.

- **Practice mindfulness meditation or other forms of relaxation.** Time and again, stress-reduction techniques have been shown to reduce craving duration and intensity. Find a method that works for you and *practice*!

- **Remember that these tips might not work immediately.** The nature of alcoholism is that it can trick you into not taking action. As soon as the craving ends (and before then, if you can) start to do the real work of recovery, which is all the things you need to do to prevent cravings in the first place, and it's what this book is all about.

Narcotic Pain Pills (for People with Chronic Pain)

The following tips are for people with chronic pain who want to cut down or eliminate their use of narcotic pain pills by managing their pain in other ways.

- **Move.** The biggest risk factor for worsening chronic pain is sitting still. Don't get frozen. Sometimes fear may get in your way, but it's absolutely critical that you get active (within the safe limits prescribed by your doctor, of course). It may seem counterintuitive, but people who move have reductions in chronic pain more than those who stay still. Not sure what activities are safe for you? Ask your doctor.

- **Sleep.** The research on sleep and chronic pain is clear: sleep deprivation worsens chronic pain. If you aren't sure how to get a good night's sleep, try these tips from the Mayo Clinic: www.mayoclinic.com/health/sleep/HQ01387. Research shows that simple actions can be more effective for insomnia than sleeping pills. Sound too good to be true? The research is in: cognitive-behavioral methods for improving sleep are as effective as pills and may be even more so in the long run.

- **Remember that narcotic pain pills can make it easier for you to feel pain in the long run.** There is a fancy medical term for this: opiate-induced hyperalgesia. What you need to know is that *your individual threshold for pain* (how bad it needs to be before you really feel it, before it bothers you) can go down with long-term exposure to narcotic pain pills. Making an effort, with your doctor's approval/assistance, to reduce or eliminate your dependence on narcotic pain pills can actually improve your pain threshold in the long haul.

- **Address the stress.** Stress has been shown time and again to worsen chronic pain. People with higher stress levels also tend to take more narcotic pain medications. Reducing your stress can make it much easier to taper off your pain medications (under a doctor's supervision, of course).

- **Connect with others.** Chronic pain support groups can really make a difference. Chapter 7 of this book explores the power of groups, and they can work for chronic pain too. There are many groups to choose from. One place to start is the American Chronic Pain Association. See www.theACPA.org for more information.

- **Do things you enjoy.** As long as they are safe for you (and your doctor can tell you whether they are), staying involved in hobbies and interests that you enjoy can reduce pain.

- **Reduce or eliminate alcohol.** Alcohol can worsen chronic pain and can interact with pain medications in a way that makes pain worse over the long haul. Also, alcohol can worsen sleep—and good sleep is critical to managing chronic pain. Finally, alcohol use can make it harder to wean yourself off narcotics.

- **Ask your doctor if you can come off narcotic pain medications.** If you can, detoxing from these medications and following the suggestions in this book can dramatically reduce or eliminate cravings for addictive pain medications.

Sugar

Too much sugar can cause many health problems, including weight gain, heart disease, diabetes, tooth decay, and depression. If you have a health condition or illness, connect with your doctor or nutritionist to make sure these tips for cutting back on sugar and dealing with sugar cravings are right for you.

- **Stop eating sugar and refined carbohydrates.** This is the hardest suggestion of all. You may go through sugar withdrawal, and it can take a couple of weeks for the cravings to calm down, although each individual craving will generally only last a few minutes. One thing is clear: sugar cravers should detox from sugar if at all possible. And white flour should be avoided at all costs. To be clear: the sugar in natural foods like fruits are fine, but the white powdery/granular stuff that looks like cocaine should be avoided—for sugar cravers it's just as addictive!

- **Get your healthy sugars from whole foods, not processed foods.** That means it's better to eat oranges than drink orange juice. The fiber will fill you up as well.

- **Eat lots of vegetables.** Six to twelve servings a day. That might sound like a lot of vegetables. Guess what? It is.

Throughout this book you've learned that dealing with cravings is much more about what you *start* doing than what you *stop* doing. If you get six to twelve servings of vegetables a day (try to include as many colors as possible: orange, green, yellow, red), your sugar cravings will diminish.

- **Eat complex carbohydrates instead of refined carbohydrates.** Whole grains like quinoa, oatmeal, whole wheat, or kamut are much better than white flour for maintaining steady insulin levels. Whole wheat is better than wheat. You may need nutritional consultation if you have conditions like gluten allergy.

- **Eat five or six small meals a day.** Sugar cravers do better with grazing than with three square meals a day.

- **Eat healthy fats, avoid unhealthy fats.** Don't be afraid of fats in your diet. Olive oil, nuts (like almonds), and avocados are great examples of healthy fats. Reminder: peanuts are not nuts, they're legumes. If you are trying to lose weight, remember that nuts need to be limited to a small handful a day.

- **Eat protein at every meal.** Proteins, especially lean proteins, can really help reduce sugar cravings.

- **Plan your meals and plan your grocery shopping.** If you can write down your goals and plans, you will be much more successful in achieving them. Never grocery shop on an empty stomach. When at the grocery store, stick to the perimeter and avoid the aisles. The outer ring is where the good stuff is.

- **Connect with others.** There are many groups (Twelve Step types and others as well) that can be helpful to sugar cravers. One example is Overeaters Anonymous. See www.overeaters anonymous.org for more information.

- **Learn from others.** For tips on healthy eating, I love www
  .fitnessandfuel-la.com/blog. They're especially good at figuring
  out how to address cravings for unhealthy foods with similar
  but healthier foods. The blog is fantastic, and the duo that
  runs it really knows what they are doing when it comes to
  making healthy choices. Their recipes are particularly great
  when it comes to sugar cravings.

Chocolate

Craving chocolate is more complex than a sugar craving. Research
suggests that it's a very specific craving, more common in women,
and not entirely explained by its sweetness or sugar content. But as
a base, the sugar suggestions in the previous section will help with
chocolate cravings. Below are some additional suggestions:

- **Plan for your premenstrual period.** Obviously, this only
  applies to women. Women crave chocolate at a much higher
  rate than men, and some research suggests that chocolate
  cravings tend to peak in the immediate premenstrual period
  and for a few days into your period.[122] Get the chocolate out
  of the house and office, and stay full with healthier foods.

- **Remember that, biologically, your craving for chocolate is
  more a craving for the sensation of eating chocolate than
  for any biological effect.** Research has shown that the sensory
  effect of chocolate (taste, texture, smell) is what you primarily
  crave, and only to a lesser extent the effects of the chemicals
  in chocolate, like xanthines. That means if the cravings are
  particularly bad, you can satisfy them with the other suggestions listed in this book, plus a small amount of sugar-free
  dark chocolate. This should be a last resort.

- **As with all cravings, wait it out.** Chocolate cravings tend to
  only last a few minutes, although they can feel like a lifetime.
  Distract yourself, call someone, eat a healthier snack, and
  follow the other suggestions in this book rather than give in.

- **Address your stress.** Stress and cravings are tightly linked, and chocolate cravings are no different. Get a handle on your stress before it gets a handle on you.

- **Take magnesium.** Ask your doctor if magnesium is safe for you, but some research suggests that chocolate cravings during a woman's premenstrual timeframe may be linked to magnesium deficiency. Chelated magnesium supplementation may help. See your doctor for the dose that's right for you. Similarly, what doctors call "unopposed estrogen" may worsen chocolate cravings. Check with your doctor about the possible role of progesterone in addressing your chocolate cravings.

- **Chocolate cravings won't hurt you.** This means that giving in to a chocolate craving, if you are not prone to binge eating, can be an acceptable option for many, as long as you can do so in a way that doesn't undermine your health and fitness goals.

Gambling

For those who are having a problem with excessive gambling, the following tips can help you quit and deal with the cravings.

- **Quit smoking.** Surprised? The research shows that gambling cravings and smoking go hand in hand. But studies have also shown that nicotine replacement therapies like lozenges and patches are safe—they don't seem to worsen gambling cravings.[123]

- **Avoid cues and triggers.** Obviously, as I've shown elsewhere in this book, you can't avoid everything that reminds you of your craving. But especially in early recovery, it's important to stay away from triggers. New research in gambling addiction shows that your eyes and your attention point very strongly toward anything gambling-related, and that those automatic (and unconscious) responses increase your cravings and the chances that you will give in.

- **Consider medications.** Although naltrexone and acamprosate (medications used for drug and alcohol addiction) are not FDA-approved for compulsive gambling, a growing body of research is showing benefit, especially for naltrexone. Ask your doctor if it's a good choice for you.

- **Use the power of the group.** As we explored in chapter 7, groups can really help when it comes to cravings. Gamblers Anonymous (GA) is a Twelve Step group that has helped many people recover from compulsive gambling. I always recommend that people who are concerned about gambling answer GA's twenty questions to learn more about the impact gambling may be having in their life. This list of twenty questions can be found on their website: www.gamblersanonymous .org. GA has a specialized system called "pressure relief" that can help you deal with gambling debts in a sane, recovery-supportive manner.

- **Let your spouse and loved ones know about Gam-Anon**, which is a Twelve Step group specifically for loved ones of gambling addicts. See www.gam-anon.org for more information.

- **Change your environment.** As with most cravings, gambling addicts are often subtly affected by their environments in ways that are hard to explain until later. If you are in a situation where you are craving to gamble, consider leaving the situation and connecting with a support person.

- **Carry only the amount of money you need for daily essentials, and don't carry checks or credit cards.** Adding barriers to accessing funds can help when the cravings hit.

- **Be accountable.** For some people with gambling addiction, temporarily having someone you absolutely trust manage your finances, and also giving a spouse or loved one access to your transactions, can be a way to remain accountable. If you ask for money or make a withdrawal without a good explanation, it can let them know you may be in trouble.

- **Address your stress.** The suggestions in the previous lists are helpful for gambling cravings as well. Sleep, stress, and mood all affect gambling cravings. Get help for them if they are a problem.

- **Set up safeguards.** Have an accountability partner block gaming sites on your computer and help you close your gaming accounts. Set up email filters to block gambling establishments and websites from contacting you, or, better yet, change your email address. If you gamble with a partner, let him know you are no longer available for gambling. If the person pressures you, he is not your real friend. Close your credit cards and put a fraud alert on your credit file, which adds an extra step you must go through to obtain credit.

- **Postpone gambling.** Remember that all cravings are short-lived. If you can distract yourself, call a friend, do something healthy and interesting, or do something that cheers you up, that can make the difference between success and relapse.

Internet Compulsions

The Internet is a wonderful thing, and most people use it without major problems. However, if you find yourself lying about your Internet use, using the Internet in secret, compromising your values when surfing online, feeling shame about your online activities, or finding yourself in a "bubble" where you stay online for hours and avoid eating, drinking, or engaging anyone else, you likely have an Internet addiction. In particular, if your relationships or work or school performance are suffering because of your Internet use, you most likely have an Internet addiction. Internet addictions can have tolerance, withdrawal, cravings, and all the major features found in other addictions.

Although not a formal diagnosis (yet), I've seen many such cases and they can be very serious. Sometimes, just as with drug addiction or alcoholism, you may need to detox completely first. Once you've been offline, it may be safe and appropriate to re-introduce Internet use by following these tips. But if you find yourself out of control again, you may need even more time off and more support. In some cases, you may need to remain completely offline; in others, not using a particular application, device, or website may be the answer. The only way to know is to try it with an accountability partner, and then see whether you need moderation or abstinence.

College students are particularly at risk, as they leave home and have large blocks of unsupervised and unstructured time and nearly unlimited access to the Internet. College counseling programs are beginning to offer support for these students. Here are some tips that can help if you think you have a problem. If moderating your use of the Internet is unsuccessful, you may need to skip these steps, get help, and stop completely.

- **Get accountable.** Allowing someone you trust to access your computer and see what you're up to can help you avoid the temptation to be swallowed up in the numb world of Internet addiction. A trusting partner who will rotate the Wi-Fi password in the home can help too. I know one mom who furnishes the daily Wi-Fi password to her kids *after* their chores and homework are done.

- **Get really accountable.** If Internet compulsion is a serious problem for you, ask your partner to hold your computer or password, and only go online with him or her present.

- **Let your laptop battery die.** Not plugging in your laptop means that the battery itself can serve as a stopwatch for the duration of your online activities.

- **Avoid cues and triggers.** Obviously, as I've shown elsewhere in this book, you can't avoid everything that reminds you of your craving. But putting your computer away is a good start.

- **Ditch the smartphone.** These days it can be hard to find a simple cell phone—but trust me, they do still exist. You'll be forced to limit the amount of time you spend online.

- **Focus on some offline relationships.** As with most compulsions, recovery from cravings is mostly about what you *start* doing and less about what you *stop* doing. Focus on doing things with a few friends in real life. Get coffee, go for a walk, get outside, or even just talk on the phone. Connect with people without using the computer as a medium, so that your brain can begin to unpair the connection between relating and being online.

- **Reconnect with your hobbies.** If you don't have any, ask your friends or family members what they like to do.

- **Try the other suggestions in this book.** For example, attend a mutual-help group for people with similar problems. Focus on helping others. Get physically active. Talk to others about your problem. Document your behaviors. You'll quickly see that the suggestions found throughout this book will apply very well to your Internet compulsions.

An additional point: most Internet and computer-related compulsions fall into one of a few categories, which I have listed here. Each type of compulsion is different and requires a specialized approach to treatment. For example, online gaming addicts may benefit from therapy for gambling addiction. Compulsive online shoppers may need to hand over their credit cards. Gamers may need to deactivate their profiles. The categories of Internet/computer-related compulsions include:

- Pornography, online dating, sexting/online flirting, chatrooms/webcams, and other forms of pseudointimacy, which may or may not be sexualized

- Gambling such as poker, sports betting, and day trading

- Shopping compulsions, eBay, etc.

- Obsessive searching/surfing, or workaholic tendencies online

- Facebook, Twitter, Pinterest, and social media-related compulsions

- Games (ranging from the immersive massive multiplayer online role-playing games such as World of Warcraft, to multiplayer games like Call of Duty, to somewhat social games such as Words with Friends and Farmville, to solo games such as Solitaire and Minesweeper)

• • •

Appendix

A Field Polarized
The Uncomfortable Gap between Cognitive Therapies and Twelve Step Programs

The cognitive view of addiction mostly derives from a classic paper by Albert Bandura (required reading for anyone studying addictions) who, in 1977, proposed that a person's expectation of self-efficacy predicts whether coping strategies will be initiated, how much effort will be expended on coping, and how resilient those efforts will be to stress and other challenges.[124] Of course, this makes sense, as you would expect that how likely you are to do something depends on how well you think it will work.

The late Alan Marlatt, considered by many to be the father of craving research, spent his career further developing and testing this idea. Marlatt proposed that whether or not an alcoholic will drink in a high-risk situation is determined by what the person believes the consequences of drinking will be. Various distortions in the alcoholic's thinking cause the person to draw erroneous conclusions about the relationship between their choices and their results. Therapies can then be targeted to address the behaviors that can land alcoholics in high-risk situations with a particular focus on the false conclusions that people draw about the relationship between certain decisions and the results. These therapies can also focus on analyzing the drinker's responses to high-risk situations and then help the alcoholic develop strategies to more effectively deal with these stressors. This increases the person's confidence that they will be successful, so that they will be more likely to expend the effort to do what's needed to stay sober in the future. Marlatt emphasized concepts such as the "covert antecedents" and "immediate determinants" of relapse, and noted that many of the decisions alcoholics make that seem irrelevant or unrelated to their drinking at the time are often directly responsible for relapse. And research does confirm that his approach can help many people with alcoholism, especially in the short term, to avoid self-destructive behaviors by interrupting and correcting the decision cycle.

According to Marlatt, when alcoholics are exposed to a high-risk situation, if their responses are ineffective, then their confidence in themselves is diminished, they drink, and then they experience a twist in their thinking (a cognitive distortion) called the abstinence violation effect and are more likely to drink again. The therapies that Marlatt and others who follow him have developed are designed to interrupt all aspects of this cascade and restore the person's sense of efficacy and the cognitive and behavioral tools in their toolbox.

FIGURE 1

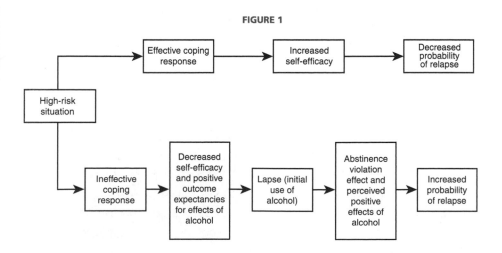

The diagram above shows how this works, and it makes a lot of sense.[125] Craving researchers have tested components of this model and found that it seems to hold up; in other words, the model does a fairly good job of explaining what happens when alcoholics cope effectively with risky situations and what happens when they don't. According to this model, self-efficacy is the key to decreasing the probability of relapse.

Unfortunately, however, this seems to be at odds with Twelve Step philosophies. That wouldn't be a big deal if Twelve Step programs weren't so effective at helping many people get and stay sober. However, these programs *are* effective, and a central tenet of their system appears to be that efficacy comes from a higher power and that the self (or, more precisely, the *ego*) is actually the source of the problem. Twelve Step programs de-emphasize the importance of self and suggest that a person himself cannot generate robust thinking to prevent the initiation of substance use.[126]

How can we resolve this apparent discrepancy? Which is it? Do alcoholics stay sober because of self-efficacy and learning new responses to high-risk situations à la Marlatt? Or do they stay sober because of admitting that they are powerless and accepting a higher power? These views are so opposed that the treatment field has not, in most cases, successfully resolved them. Instead, the field of addiction treatment has been polarized, with Twelve Step camps over here and cognitive-behavioral therapists over there, and "never the twain shall meet." Although there are many exceptions, the trend has been for academics to be on the cognitive (or related) side, and nonacademics to be more Twelve Step biased.

The problem is not, however, simply a theoretical one or simply academic. Patients have suffered from the confusion and mixed messaging. After all, AA and other Twelve Step programs are based on the idea that a higher power can do what the individual cannot. Since many patients who enroll in treatment programs that espouse Marlatt's approach will learn that self-efficacy is paramount to sobriety, their success may be undermined when they attend Twelve Step meetings and learn that the self is the problem and that only a higher power can keep them sober. I have been observing this dynamic for over a decade, and I can tell you that it is the source of much confusion, heartache, and even relapse.

Part of the confusion is over the term "self-efficacy." The term "self" is both unnecessary and unnecessarily confusing. If we think of this as simply efficacy (rather than self-efficacy), much of the debate dissolves. Long-sober Twelve Step program members describe an unshakable faith that their participation in these pro- grams will produce recovery. They know the Twelve Step program works. This sense of efficacy (although not exactly *self*-efficacy) drives their results in just the way Bandura and Marlatt predicted. True, they attribute their success to a power greater than themselves. Most, however, accept the notion that the power resides deep within themselves, although they emphasize that it is not the same as them- selves.[127] Seen this way, Marlatt's diagram is highly consistent with Twelve Step views, including the experience that a series of actions (the Steps), when taken, render the sufferer able to cope effectively with high-risk situations.

Another difference between talk therapies for addictive disorders and Twelve Step methodologies (leaving aside the obvious differ- ence that Twelve Step programs are not therapy, although there are therapies that are specifically designed to facilitate Twelve Step participation) is that, in general, Twelve Step programs emphasize that they are designed to help those people who want to stop using alcohol (or the drug or other problem behavior). True, many people attend Twelve Step meetings before they are ready to stop (and that can often be helpful for some ambivalent people), but the programs are generally pretty clear about who they are designed to help— those who want it. Consider these lines from the book *Alcoholics Anonymous*, fourth edition:

> "We are assuming, of course, that the reader desires to
> stop." (p. 34)

"If you have decided you want what we have and are willing to go to any lengths to get it—then you are ready to take certain steps." (p. 58)

Cognitive therapies and similar methods (including one called Motivational Enhancement Therapy) can be used for people who are not yet ready to stop. Or, simply put, treatment is about *dis*-covery and Twelve Step programs are about *re*-covery. So another key difference between these methods is the appropriate target population.

Yet another source of disagreement (or confusion) stems from the erroneous notion that Twelve Step programs tell you that you cannot think your way out of a drink (or a drug, or an addictive behavior), whereas cognitive methods such as Marlatt's emphasize thinking (and improving the thinking process, if you will, via certain therapies) as a critical solution to high-risk situations. Well, which is it? Can you think your way to sobriety or can't you? What is the role of thinking, and which camp is correct? Once again, although many in the field haven't been able to see this clearly, the views aren't really so opposed. In fact, Twelve Step programs emphasize the importance of thinking, once the dysfunctional thinking patterns have been addressed using the Twelve Steps:

On awakening let us think about the twenty-four hours ahead. We consider our plans for the day. Before we begin, we ask God to direct our thinking, especially asking that it be divorced from self-pity, dishonest or self-seeking motives. Under these conditions we can employ our mental faculties with assurance, for after all God gave us brains to use. Our thought-life will be placed on a much higher plane when our thinking is cleared of wrong motives.[128]

In other words, both the cognitive approach to managing cravings and the Twelve Step methods emphasize that dysfunctional thinking (described in *Alcoholics Anonymous* as mental obsession, delusion, or wrong-motive thinking) drives alcoholic behavior and that transformative experiences are required to address that. In his later years, Marlatt became involved in developing mindfulness-based therapies to reduce cravings and substance use, which are very closely related to Twelve Step approaches.

I don't mean to suggest that these philosophies are identical—they aren't at all. Twelve Step programs emphasize the absolute importance of recognizing that there is a power greater than the individual and the importance of relying on that power in everything they do. Cognitive and related therapies emphasize the absolute importance of changing the way we think, through exercises that force us to examine and alter distortions in the conclusions about the facts of our experience. My point is that they really aren't mutually exclusive and that more could be done for people who benefit from cognitive methods to help them incorporate Twelve Step programs into their recoveries without creating such a drastic (and destructive) either/or. This is important, because much of the psychosocial support available to people who suffer from cravings can be found in Twelve Step fellowships, and it can be much easier to access the key ingredients of successful recovery by utilizing these programs.

The bottom line is this: in the throes of addictive disease, and in the midst of craving, people will not always be able to rely on their brains to help them avoid succumbing to their urges. They may *sometimes* be able to use their thinking to help them, but for anyone who wants consistent success, something more is needed. Their thinking needs to change; *they* need to change. That requires actions of the type that I'm describing in this book.

. . .

Notes

1. John M. Harlow, "Recovery from the Passage of an Iron Bar through the Head," *History of Psychiatry* 4, no. 14 (1993): 274–81.

2. J. P. Brasil-Neto, A. Pascual-Leone, J. Valls-Sole, L. G. Cohen, and M. Hallett, "Focal Transcranial Magnetic Stimulation and Response Bias in a Forced-Choice Task," *Journal of Neurology, Neurosurgery & Psychiatry* 55, no. 10 (October 1992): 964–66.

3. S. Fecteau, A. Pascual-Leone, D. H. Zald, P. Liguori, H. Theoret, P. S. Boggio, and F. Fregni, "Activation of Prefrontal Cortex by Transcranial Direct Current Stimulation Reduces Appetite for Risk During Ambiguous Decision Making," *Journal of Neuroscience* 27, no. 23 (2007): 6212–18.

4. These results were presented in December 2011 at the Neural Information Processing Systems' Machine Learning and Interpretation in Neuroimaging workshop in Sierra Nevada, Spain.

5. R. Verheul, W. van den Brink, and P. Geerlings, "A Three-Pathway Psychological Model of Craving for Alcohol," *Alcohol and Alcoholism* 34 (1999): 197–222.

6. James Olds and Peter Milner, "Positive Reinforcement Produced by Electrical Stimulation of the Septal Area and Other Regions of Rat Brain," *Journal of Comparative and Physiological Psychology* 47, no. 6 (1954): 419–27.

7. In 1998, Dr. Lynn Churchill from Washington State University demonstrated that the brain's connections *actually reorganize* in response to reduced dopamine, resulting in changes in the way opiates affect motor activity. This is just one of many examples of how the brain's connections adapt and change in response to decreased (and increased) dopamine.

8. Nassima Ait-Daoud, John D. Roache, Michael A. Dawes, Lei Liu, Xin-Qun Wang, Martin A. Javors, Chamindi Seneviratne, and Bankole A. Johnson, "Can Serotonin Transporter Genotype Predict Craving in Alcoholism?" *Alcoholism: Clinical & Experimental Research* 33, no. 8 (2009): 1329–35.

9. For a nice review of the relationship between serotonin and alcoholism, see David LeMarquanda, Robert O. Pihl, and Chawki Benkelfat, "Serotonin and Alcohol Intake, Abuse, and Dependence: Clinical Evidence," *Biological Psychiatry* 36, no. 5 (1994): 326–37.

10. P. Huttnen and R. D. Myers, "Anatomical Localization in Hippocampus of Tetrahydro-Beta-Carboline Induced Alcohol Drinking in the Rat," *Alcohol* 4, no. 3 (1987): 181–87.

11. For a more detailed review of this hypothesis, see K. Blum, E. R. Braverman, J. M. Holder, J. F. Lubar, V. J. Monastra, D. Miller, J. O. Lubar, T. J. Chen, and D. E. Comings, "Reward Deficiency Syndrome: A Biogenetic Model for the Diagnosis and Treatment of Impulsive, Addictive, and Compulsive Behaviors," *Journal of Psychoactive Drugs* 32, Suppl. i–iv (2000): 1–112.

12. For a great review of this and other theories, see Giovanni Addolorato, Lorenzo Leggio, Ludovico Abenavoli, Giovanni Gasbarrini on behalf of the Alcoholism Treatment Study Group, "Neurobiochemical and Clinical Aspects of Craving in Alcohol Addiction: A Review," *Addictive Behaviors* 30 (2005): 1209–24.

13. Alec Horniman is the Killgallon Ohio Art Professor of Business Administration and a Senior Fellow of the Olsson Center for Applied Ethics. He teaches ethics, strategy, and leadership at the Darden Graduate School of Business at the University of Virginia.

14. Rachel L. Goldman, Jeffrey J. Borckardt, Heather A. Frohman, Patrick M. O'Neil, Alok Madan, Laura K. Campbell, Amanda Budak, and Mark S. George, "Prefrontal Cortex Transcranial Direct Current Stimulation (TDCS) Temporarily Reduces Food Cravings and Increases the Self-Reported Ability to Resist Food in Adults with Frequent Food Craving," *Appetite* 56, no. 3 (2011): 741–46.

15. J. M. Bossert, A. L. Stern, F. R. Theberge, C. Cifani, E. Koya, B. T. Hope, and Y. Shaham, "Ventral Medial Prefrontal Cortex Neuronal Ensembles Mediate Context-Induced Relapse to Heroin," *Nature Neuroscience* 14 (2011): 420–22.

16. Marika Tiggemann, Eva Kemps, and Jasmin Parnell, "The Selective Impact of Chocolate Craving on Visuospatial Working Memory," *Appetite* 55, no. 1 (2010): 44–48.

17. R. Suñer-Soler, A. Grau, M. E. Gras, S. Font-Mayolas, Y. Silva, A. Dávalos, V. Cruz, J. Rodrigo, and J. Serena, "Smoking Cessation 1 Year Poststroke and Damage to the Insular Cortex," *Stroke* 43, no. 1 (2012): 131–36. Epub Nov. 3, 2011.

18. S. A. McKee, R. Sinha, A. H. Weinberger, M. Sofuoglu, E. L. Harrison, M. Lavery, and J. Wanzer, "Stress Decreases the Ability to Resist Smoking and Potentiates Smoking Intensity and Reward," *Journal of Psychopharmacology* 25, no. 4 (2011): 490–502.

19. H. C. Fox, K. A. Hong, and R. Sinha, "Difficulties in Emotion Regulation and Impulse Control in Recently Abstinent Alcoholics Compared with Social Drinkers," *Addictive Behaviors* 33, no. 2 (2008): 388–94.

20. K. Grasing, D. Mathur, and C. Desouza, "Written Emotional Expression during Recovery from Cocaine Dependence: Group and Individual Differences in Craving Intensity," *Substance Use and Misuse* 45, no. 7–8 (2010): 1201–15.

21. In fact, in 2007 Hilke Plassman and colleagues conducted fascinating experiments to determine how much hungry subjects were willing to pay for various foods. These ingenious experiments using brain imaging confirmed that activity in the subjects' orbitofrontal cortex and dorsolateral prefrontal cortex (which are parts of the prefrontal cortex) is responsible for determining these subjects' willingness to pay. In recovery, including in AA and other Twelve Step programs, willingness is emphasized as essential to taking the necessary actions that result in behavioral and spiritual transformation. It seems that the willingness to take actions that result in improvement in our lives is at least, in part, prefrontally driven.

22. The etymology of the word "crave" suggests that it is derived from the Old English "crafian," to demand. In most cases where cravings are concerning or problematic for my patients, they don't describe them as requests, but rather as necessities; "demand" seems about right.

23. AA World Services, *Alcoholics Anonymous,* 4th ed. (New York: AA World Services, 1991), chapter 3.

24. The largest study to address this question has been Project MATCH. This group concluded that more severe alcoholics (those, for example, who require inpatient treatment) fare better with Twelve Step approaches than cognitive-behavioral approaches. This suggests that the more severe the craving, the less likely you will be able to think your way out of it.

25. In fact, AA is more widely used than any other method to address alcohol addiction; C. Weisner, T. Greenfiels, and R. Room, "Trends in the Treatment of Alcohol Problems in the U.S. General Population, 1979 through 1990," *American Journal of Public Health* 85, no. 1 (1995): 55–60.

26. For a fascinating look at the ways you can trick yourself into believing you have achieved insight, see David McRaney, *You Are Not So Smart: Why You Have Too Many Friends on Facebook, Why Your Memory Is Mostly Fiction,* and *46 Other Ways You're Deluding Yourself* (New York: Dutton, 2011). McRaney describes in simple language many of the ways your mind fools you into believing things that aren't true and why it's important that your mind does that.

27. Akitoshi Ogawa, Yumiko Yamazaki, Kenichi Ueno, Kang Cheng, and Atsushi Iriki, "Neural Correlates of Species-Typical Illogical Cognitive Bias in Human Inference," *Journal of Cognitive Neuroscience* 22, no. 9 (2010): 2120–30.

28. This is from the work of Jochen Musch from the University of Mannheim. "Personality Differences in Hindsight Bias," *Memory* 11, no. 4–5 (2003): 473–89.

29. Wolfgang Hell, Gerd Gigerenzer, Siegfried Gauggel, Maria Mall, and Michael Muller, "Hindsight Bias: An Interaction of Automatic and Motivational Factors?" *Memory & Cognition* 16, no. 6 (1988): 533–38.

30. Britta Renner, "Hindsight Bias after Receiving Self-Relevant Health Risk Information: A Motivational Perspective," *Memory* 11, no. 4–5 (2003): 455–72.

31. Emily Pronin, Justin Kruger, Kenneth Savitsky, and Lee Ross, "You Don't Know Me, But I Know You: The Illusion of Asymmetric Insight," *Journal of Personality and Social Psychology* 81, no. 4 (2001): 639–56.

32. Thomas Shelley Duval and Paul J. Silvia, "Self-Awareness, Probability of Improvement, and the Self-Serving Bias," *Journal of Personality & Social Psychology* 82, no. 1 (2002): 49–61.

33. Joyce Ehrlinger, Thomas Gilovich, and Lee Ross, "Peering into the Bias Blind Spot: People's Assessments of Bias in Themselves and Others," *Personality & Social Psychology Bulletin* 31, no. 5 (2005): 680–92.

34. R. E. Meyer and S. M. Mirin, *The Heroin Stimulus: Implications for a Theory of Addiction* (New York: Plenum, 1979).

35. Paul D. Cherulnik and Murray M. Citrin, "Individual Difference in Psychological Reactance: The Interaction Between Locus of Control and Mode of Elimination of Freedom," *Journal of Personality and Social Psychology* 29, no. 3 (1974): 398–404.

36. AA World Services, "The Doctor's Opinion," *Alcoholics Anonymous,* xxv.

37. John Bradshaw, *Healing the Shame That Binds You* (Deerfield Beach, FL: Health Communications Inc., 2005), 136.

38. Thomas J. Scheff, UCSB website, www.soc.ucsb.edu/faculty/scheff/main .php?id=2.html.

39. L. E. O'Connor and colleagues demonstrated this several years ago when they measured shame, detachment, and depression in recovering addicts, some of whom were still in residential treatment and some of whom were in active recovery in Twelve Step fellowships. Compared to nonaddicted people, recovering addicts were much more prone to shame (and less prone to guilt), and women were more likely to exhibit shame overtly whereas men were more likely to show signs of emotional detachment. L. E. O'Connor, J. W. Berry, D. Inaba, J. Weiss, and A. Morrison, "Shame, Guilt, and Depression in Men and Women in Recovery from Addiction," *Journal of Substance Abuse Treatment* 11, no. 6 (1994): 503–10.

40. For an excellent review of shame and addiction from an academic perspective, see Shelly Wiechelt's review "The Specter of Shame" in *Substance Use & Misuse* 42, no. 2–3 (2007): 399–409.

41. Marc Schuckit, "Genetics of the Risk for Alcoholism," *American Journal on Addictions* 9, no. 2 (2000): 103–12.

42. L. J. Bierut, S. H. Dinwiddie, H. Begleiter, R. R. Crowe, V. Hesselbrock, J. I. Nurnberger Jr., B. Porjesz, M. A. Schuckit, and T. Reich, "Familial Transmission of Substance Dependence: Alcohol, Marijuana, Cocaine, and Habitual Smoking: A Report from the Collaborative Study on the Genetics of Alcoholism," *Archives of General Psychiatry* 55, no. 11 (1998): 982–88.

43. AA World Services, *The AA Member—Medications and Other Drugs* (New York: AA World Services, 2011). Of note, this pamphlet was written by physicians in recovery from alcoholism.

44. Michael A. Sayette, Christopher S. Martin, Joan M. Wertz, Michael A. Perrott, and Annie R. Peters, "The Effects of Alcohol on Cigarette Craving in Heavy Smokers and Tobacco Chippers," *Psychology of Addictive Behaviors* 19, no. 3 (2005): 263–70.

45. American Psychiatric Association, *Diagnostic and Statistical Manual of Mental Disorders*, DSM-IV-TR, Fourth Edition (Text Revision) (New York: American Psychiatric Publishing, 2000).

46. L. F. Fontenelle, S. Oostermeijer, B. J. Harrison, C. Pantelis, and M. Yücel, "Obsessive-Compulsive Disorder, Impulse Control Disorders and Drug Addiction Common Features and Potential Treatments," *Drugs* 71, no. 7 (2011): 827–40.

47. For a very nice review of the similarities between these conditions and more detail on the imaging and neurochemical similarities between these conditions, see Leonardo Fontenelle's paper cited above.

48. J. E. Grant, "Family History and Psychiatric Comorbidity in Persons with Kleptomania," *Comprehensive Psychiatry* 44, no. 6 (2003): 437–41.

49. Specifically, both kleptomania and cocaine addiction show decreased white matter microstructural integrity in the ventral-medial frontal brain regions compared to controls.

50. Jon E. Grant, Brian L. Odlaug, and SuckWon Kim, "Kleptomania: Clinical Characteristics and Relationship to Substance Use Disorders," *American Journal of Drug and Alcohol Abuse* 36, no. 5 (2010): 291–95.

51. Marc N. Potenza, "The Neurobiology of Pathological Gambling and Drug Addiction: An Overview and New Findings," *Philosophical Transactions of the Royal Society of London. Series B, Biological Sciences* 363 (2008): 3181–89.

52. All of these findings are very well reviewed by Jon Grant from the University of Minnesota, in Jon E. Grant, Judson A. Brewer, and Marc N. Potenza, "The Neurobiology of Substance and Behavioral Addictions," *CNS Spectrums* 11, no. 12 (2006): 924–30.

53. J. Gunstad, R. H. Paul, R. A. Cohen, D. F. Tate, M. B. Spitznagel, and E. Gordon, "Elevated Body Mass Index Is Associated with Executive Dysfunction in Otherwise Healthy Adults," *Comprehensive Psychiatry* 48, no. 1 (2007): 57–61.

54. Nora D. Volkow, Gene-Jack Wang, Frank Telang, Joanna S. Fowler, Rita Z. Goldstein, Nelly Alia-Klein, Jean Logan, Christopher Wong, Panayotis K. Thanos, Yemine Ma, and Kith Pradhan, "Inverse Association between BMI and Prefrontal Metabolic Activity in Healthy Adults," *Obesity* 17, no. 1 (2009): 60–65.

55. Sakura Komatsu, "Rice and Sushi Cravings: A Preliminary Study of Food Craving among Japanese Females," *Appetite* 50, no. 2–3 (2008): 353–58.

56. Mark Griffiths, professor at Nottingham Trent University, has published a very useful tool to help practitioners screen for these disorders by looking for precisely these symptoms. M. D. Griffiths, A. Szabo, and A. Terry, "The Exercise Addiction Inventory: A Quick and Easy Screening Tool for Health Practitioners," *British Journal of Sports Medicine* 39, no. 6 (2005): e30.

57. These aspects of exercise dependence are well reviewed by Ian Cockerill and Megan Riddington, "Exercise Dependence and Associated Disorders: A Review," *Counselling Psychology Quarterly* 9, no. 2 (1996): 119–29.

58. M. Varvel, "Exercise Addiction: An Examination of Associated Personality Characteristics" (unpublished dissertation, School of Sport and Exercise Sciences, University of Birmingham, 1992).

59. Den'etsu Sutoo and Kayo Akiyama, "Regulation of Brain Function by Exercise," *Neurobiology of Disease* 13, no. 1 (2003): 1–14.

60. A. Yates, C. Shisslak, M. Crago, and J. Allender, "Overcommitment to Sport: Is There a Relationship to the Eating Disorders?" *Clinical Journal of Sport Medicine* 4, no. 1 (1994): 39–46.

61. Michel Reynaud, Laurent Karila, Lisa Blecha, and Amine Benyamina, "Is Love Passion an Addictive Disorder?" *The American Journal of Drug and Alcohol Abuse* 36, no. 5 (2010): 261–67.

62. Michel Reynaud, Laurent Karila, Lisa Blecha, and Amine Benyamina, "Is Love Passion an Addictive Disorder?" *The American Journal of Drug and Alcohol Abuse* 36, no. 5 (2010): 261–67.

63. Mary-Frances O'Connor, David K. Wellisch, Annette L. Stanton, Naomi I. Eisenberger, Michael R. Irwin, and Matthew D. Lieberman, "Craving Love? Enduring Grief Activates Brain's Reward Center," *Neuroimage* 42, no. 2 (2008): 969–72.

64. *Welcome to Narcotics Anonymous* by Narcotics Anonymous World Services, Inc., 1986. See www.na.org/admin/include/spaw2/uploads/pdf/litfiles /us_english/IP/EN3122.pdf.

65. S. J. Blatt, B. Rounsaville, S. L. Eyre, and C. Wilber, "The Psychodynamics of Opiate Addiction," *Journal of Nervous & Mental Disease* 172, no. 6 (1984): 342–52.

66. G. O. Gabbard, *Psychodynamic Psychiatry in Clinical Practice* (Arlington, VA: American Psychiatric Publishing, 2005).

67. The other major problem that impairs outcomes is that although addictions are chronic diseases, most of our systems of care are designed to treat them in an acute fashion. This mismatch is also a contributor to the poor outcomes we sometimes see in addiction treatment. Emphasis on ongoing recovery support, often termed "recovery management," is a key to long-term success.

68. A. D. Pellegrini and P. D. Davis, "Relations between Children's Playground and Classroom Behavior," *British Journal of Educational Psychology* 63, no. 1 (1993): 88–95.

69. Jaakko Mursu, Kim Robien, Lisa J. Harnack, Kyong Park, and David R. Jacobs Jr., "Dietary Supplements and Mortality Rate in Older Women: The Iowa Women's Health Study," *Archives of Internal Medicine* 171, no. 18 (2011): 1625–33.

70. M. J. Eckardt and P. R. Martin, "Clinical Assessment of Cognition in Alcoholism," *Alcoholism: Clinical and Experimental Research* 10, no. 2 (1986): 123–27.

71. H. Franke, H. Kittner, P. Berger, K. Wirkner, and J. Schramek, "The Reaction of Astrocytes and Neurons in the Hippocampus of Adult Rats during Chronic Ethanol Treatment and Correlations to Behavioral Impairments," *Alcohol* 14, no. 5 (1997): 445–54.

72. For more on this, see Steven Casper's fascinating blog, www.dictionary ofneurology.com.

73. A. Pascual-Leone, D. Nguyet, L. G. Cohen, J. P. Brasil-Neto, A. Cammarota, and M. Hallett, "Modulation of Muscle Responses Evoked by Transcranial Magnetic Stimulation during the Acquisition of New Fine Motor Skills," *Journal of Neurophysiology* 74, no. 3 (1995): 1037–45.

74. Valerie A. Cardenas, Kristin Samuelson, Maryann Lenoci, Colin Studholme, Thomas C. Neylan, Charles R. Marmar, Norbert Schuff, and Michael W. Weiner, "Changes in Brain Anatomy during the Course of Posttraumatic Stress Disorder," *Psychiatry Research* 193, no. 2 (2011): 93–100.

75. K. Goldapple, Z. Segal, C. Garson, M. Lau, P. Bieling, S. Kennedy, and H. S. Mayberg, "Modulation of Cortical-Limbic Pathways in Major Depression: Treatment-Specific Effects of CBT," *Archives of General Psychiatry* 61, no. 1 (2004): 34–41.

76. R. J. Davidson and A. Lutz, "Buddha's Brain: Neuroplasticity and Meditation," *IEEE Signal Processing Magazine* 25, no. 1 (2008): 171–74.

77. Benedetto De Martino, D. Kumaran, B. Seymour, and R. J. Dolan, "Frames, Biases, and Rational Decision-Making in the Human Brain," *Science* 313, no. 5787 (2006): 684–87.

78. K. N. Javaras, S. M. Schaefer, C. M. van Reekum, R. C. Lapate, L. L. Greischar, D. R. Bachhuber, G. Dienberg Love, C. D. Ryff, and R. J. Davidson, "Conscientiousness Predicts Greater Recovery from Negative Emotion," *Emotion* 12, no. 5 (2012): 875–81.

79. Stanley Colcombe and Arthur F. Kramer, "Fitness Effects on the Cognitive Function of Older Adults: A Meta-Analytic Study," *Psychological Science* 14, no. 2 (2003).

80. Bill Wilson, "Spiritus contra Spiritum: The Bill Wilson/C. G. Jung Letters: The Roots of the Society of Alcoholics Anonymous," *Parabola* 12, no. 2 (May 1987): 68–69.

81. J. S. Tonigan, W. R. Miller, and G. J. Connors, "The Search for Meaning in Life as a Predictor of Alcoholism Treatment Outcome," in *Project MATCH Hypotheses: Results and Causal Chain Analyses.* Project MATCH Monograph Series, vol. 8., ed. R. Longabaugh and P. W. Wirtz (Bethesda, MD: National Institute on Alcohol Abuse and Alcoholism, 2001), 154–65.

82. H. G. Koenig, L. K. George, K. G. Meador, D. G. Blazer, and S. M. Ford, "Religious Practices and Alcoholism in a Southern Adult Population," *Hospital & Community Psychiatry* 45, no. 3 (1994): 225–31.

83. Sat Bir S. Khalsa, Gurucharan S. Khalsa, Hargopal K. Khalsa, and Mukta K. Khalsa, "Evaluation of a Residential Kundalini Yoga Lifestyle Pilot Program for Addiction in India," *Journal of Ethnicity in Substance Abuse* 7, no. 1 (2008): 67–79.

84. Wahiba Abu-Ras, Sameera Ahmed, and Cynthia L. Arfken, "Alcohol Use among U.S. Muslim College Students: Risk and Protective Factors," *Journal of Ethnicity in Substance Abuse* 9, no. 3 (2010): 206–20.

85. C. Timko, R. H. Moos, J. W. Finney, and M. D. Lesar, "Long-Term Outcomes of Alcohol Use Disorders: Comparing Untreated Individuals with Those in Alcoholics Anonymous and Formal Treatment," *Journal of Studies on Alcohol and Drugs* 61, no. 4 (2000): 529–40.

86. S. R. Walker, J. S. Tonigan, W. R. Miller, S. Corner, and L. Kahlich, "Intercessory Prayer in the Treatment of Alcohol Abuse and Dependence: A Pilot Investigation," *Alternative Therapies in Health and Medicine* 3, no. 6 (1997): 79–86.

87. See especially K. Piderman, T. Schneekloth, V. Pankratz, S. Maloney, and S. Altchuler, "Spirituality in Alcoholics during Treatment," *American Journal on Addictions* 6, no. 3 (2007): 232–37.

88. C. Emrick, J. Tonigan, H. Montgomery, and L. Little, "Alcoholics Anonymous: What Is Currently Known?" in *Research on Alcoholics Anonymous,* ed. B. McCrady (New Brunswick, NJ: Rutgers Center for Alcohol Studies, 1993), 41–76.

89. K. Humphreys, R. H. Moos, and C. Cohen, "Social and Community Resources and Long-Term Recovery from Treated and Untreated Alcoholism," *Journal of Studies on Alcohol* 58 (1997): 231–38.

90. R. G. Atkins Jr. and J. E. Hawdon, "Religiosity and Participation in Mutual-Aid Support Groups for Addiction," *Journal of Substance Abuse Treatment* 33, no. 3 (2007): 321–31.

91. The particular tobacco use log I'm referring to is copyrighted by the Regents of the University of California and can be found at the University of California, San Francisco Rx for Change program: http://rxforchange.ucsf.edu.

92. Katie Witkiewitz and Sarah Bowen, "Depression, Craving, and Substance Use Following a Randomized Trial of Mindfulness-Based Relapse Prevention," *Journal of Consulting & Clinical Psychology* 78, no. 3 (June 2010): 362–74.

93. Kevin W. Chen, Anthony Comerford, Phillip Shinnick, and Douglas M. Ziedonis, "Introducing Qigong Meditation into Residential Addiction Treatment: A Pilot Study Where Gender Makes a Difference," *Journal of Alternative & Complementary Medicine* 16, no. 8 (2010): 875–82.

94. B. S. Musterman, *Reptiles on Caffeine* (Cornelius, NC: Warren Publishing, 2008).

95. For a great review of the various benefits of helpfulness to cravings and addictive behaviors, see Sarah E. Zemore and Maria E. Pagano, "Kickbacks from Helping Others: Health and Recovery," *Recent Developments in Alcoholism* 18 (2008): 141–66.

96. S. G. Post, "Altruism, Happiness, and Health: It's Good to Be Good," *International Journal of Behavioral Medicine* 12, no. 2 (2005): 66–77.

97. Stephen G. Post, "It's Good to Be Good: 2011 Fifth Annual Scientific Report on Health, Happiness and Helping Others," *International Journal of Person Centered Medicine* 1, no. 4 (2011).

98. www.stephengpost.com/hiddengifts

99. K. I. Hunter and M. W. Linn, "Psychosocial Differences between Elderly Volunteers and Non-Volunteers," *International Journal of Aging and Human Development* 12 (1981): 205–13.

100. J. Webb and K. Brewer, "Forgiveness, Health, and Problematic Drinking among College Students in Southern Appalachia," *Journal of Health Psychology* 15, no. 8 (2010): 1257–66.

101. J. R. Webb, E. A. R. Robinson, and K. J. Brower, "Forgiveness and Mental Health among People Entering Outpatient Treatment with Alcohol Problems," *Alcoholism Treatment Quarterly* 27, no. 4 (2009): 368–88.

102. http://summaries.cochrane.org/CD001007/do-group-based-smoking-cessation-programmes-help-people-to-stop-smoking

103. J. Bond, L. A. Kaskutas, and C. Weisner, "The Persistent Influence of Social Networks and Alcoholics Anonymous on Abstinence," *Journal of Studies on Alcohol* 64, no. 4 (2003): 579–88. See also L. A. Kaskutas, J. Bond, and K. Humphreys, "Social Networks as Mediators of the Effect of Alcoholics Anonymous," *Addiction* 97, no. 7 (2002): 891–900.

104. John F. Kelly, Robert L. Stout, Molly Magill, and J. Scott Tonigan, "The Role of Alcoholics Anonymous in Mobilizing Adaptive Social Network Changes: A Prospective Lagged Mediational Analysis," *Drug & Alcohol Dependence* 114, no. 2–3 (2011): 119–26.

105. H. G. Roozen, R. de Waart, and P. van der Kroft, "Community Reinforcement and Family Training: An Effective Option to Engage Treatment-Resistant Substance-Abusing Individuals in Treatment," *Addiction* 105, no. 10 (Oct. 2010): 1729–38.

106. M. Galanter, *Network Therapy for Alcohol and Drug Abuse* (New York: Basic Books, 1993).

107. R. E. Meyer, "Conditioning Phenomena and the Problem of Relapse in Opioid Addicts and Alcoholics," in *Learning Factors in Substance Abuse*, ed. B. Ray, NIDA research monograph series no. 84 (1988): 61–79.

108. Reuven Dar, Nurit Rosen-Korakin, Oren Shapira, Yair Gottlieb, and Hanan Frenk, "The Craving to Smoke in Flight Attendants: Relations with Smoking Deprivation, Anticipation of Smoking, and Actual Smoking," *Journal of Abnormal Psychology* 119, no. 1 (2010): 248–53.

109. Nicole K. Lee, Sonja Pohlman, Amanda Baker, Jason Ferris, and Frances Kay-Lambkin, "It's the Thought That Counts: Craving Metacognitions and Their Role in Abstinence from Methamphetamine Use," *Journal of Substance Abuse Treatment* 38 (2010): 245–50.

110. Gantt P. Galloway, Edward G. Singleton, Raymond Buscemi, Matthew J. Baggott, Rene M. Dickerhoof, and John E. Mendelson, "An Examination of Drug Craving Over Time in Abstinent Methamphetamine Users," *American Journal on Addictions* 19, no. 6 (2010): 510–14.

111. John Hughes, "Craving among Long-Abstinent Smokers: An Internet Survey," *Nicotine & Tobacco Research* 12, no. 4 (2010): 459–62.

112. Brian L. Carter, Cho Y. Lam, Jason D. Robinson, Megan M. Paris, Andrew J. Waters, David W. Wetter, and Paul M. Cinciripini, "Generalized Craving, Self-Report of Arousal, and Cue Reactivity after Brief Abstinence," *Nicotine & Tobacco Research* 11, no. 7 (2009): 823–26.

113. Barbel Knauper, Rowena Pillay, Julien Lacaille, Amanda McCollam, and Evan Kelso, "Replacing Craving Imagery with Alternative Pleasant Imagery Reduces Craving Intensity," *Appetite* 57, no. 1 (2011): 173–78; J. May, J. Andrade, N. Panabokke, and D. Kavanagh, "Visuospatial Tasks Suppress Craving for Cigarettes," *Behaviour Research & Therapy* 48, no. 6 (2010): 476–85.

114. For a fantastic review of mindfulness-based relapse prevention, see *Mindfulness-Based Relapse Prevention for Addictive Behaviors: A Clinician's Guide* by Sarah Bowen, Neha Chawla, and G. Alan Marlatt (Guilford Press, 2010).

115. Nora D. Volkow, Joanna S. Fowler, Gene-Jack Wang, Frank Telang, Jean Logan, Millard Jayne, Yeming Ma, Kith Pradhan, Christopher Wong, and James M. Swanson, "Cognitive Control of Drug Craving Inhibits Brain Reward Regions in Cocaine Abusers," *Neuroimage* 49, no. 3 (2010): 2536–43.

116. Maciej S. Buchowski, Natalie N. Meade, Evonne Charboneau, Sohee Park, Mary S. Dietrich, Ronald L. Cowan, and Peter R. Martin, "Aerobic Exercise Training Reduces Cannabis Craving and Use in Non-Treatment Seeking Cannabis-Dependent Adults," *PLoS ONE* 6, no. 3 (2011): e17465.

117. Giovanni Martinotti, Daniela Reina, Marco Di Nicola, Sara Andreoli, Daniela Tedeschi, Ilaria Ortolani, Gino Pozzi, Emerenziana Iannoni, Stefania D'Iddio, and Luigi Janiri, "Acetyl-L-Carnitine for Alcohol Craving and Relapse Prevention in Anhedonic Alcoholics: A Randomized, Double-Blind, Placebo-Controlled Pilot Trial," *Alcohol & Alcoholism* 45, no. 5 (2010): 449–55.

118. John F. Kelly, Maria E. Pagano, Robert L. Stout, and Shannon M. Johnson, "Influence of Religiosity on 12-Step Participation and Treatment Response Among Substance-Dependent Adolescents," *Journal of Studies on Alcohol and Drugs* 72 (2011): 1000–11.

119. AA Guidelines for AA Members Employed in the Alcoholism Field, see www.aa.org/en_pdfs/mg-10_foraamembers.pdf.

120. AA World Services, *Alcoholics Anonymous,* 77.

121. Ernest Kurtz, *Spirituality of Imperfection: Storytelling and the Search for Meaning* (New York: Bantam Books, 2002), 20.

122. Paul Rozin, Eleanor Levine, and Caryn Stoess, "Chocolate Craving and Liking," *Appetite* 17, no. 3 (1991): 199–212.

123. D. S. McGrath, S. P. Barrett, S. H. Stewart, and E. A. Schmid, "The Effects of Acute Doses of Nicotine on Video Lottery Terminal Gambling in Daily Smokers," *Psychopharmacology* 220, no. 1 (March 2012): 155–61.

124. Albert Bandura, "Self-Efficacy: Toward a Unifying Theory of Behavioral Change," *Psychological Review* 84, no. 2 (March 1977): 191–215.

125. Mary E. Larimer, Rebekka S. Palmer, and G. Alan Marlatt, "Relapse Prevention: An Overview of Marlatt's Cognitive-Behavioral Model," *Alcohol Research & Health* 23, no. 2 (1999).

126. AA World Services, *Alcoholics Anonymous,* 43. "Once more: The alcoholic at certain times has no effective mental defense against the first drink. . . . [N]either he nor any other human being can provide such a defense. His defense must come from a Higher Power."

127. *Alcoholics Anonymous,* 55. "We found the Great Reality deep down within us. In the last analysis, it is only there that He may be found." [underlining mine].

128. *Alcoholics Anonymous,* 86.

About the Author

Omar Manejwala, M.D., is a psychiatrist and an internationally recognized expert on addiction and compulsive behavior. He is the former medical director of Hazelden, a treatment center in Center City, Minnesota, and currently the chief medical officer of Catasys, a health management services company specializing in substance dependence. He has appeared on numerous national media programs including *20/20, CBS Evening News,* and *The Early Show.* Although he is an expert on craving, he hasn't yet conquered his own craving for spending time with his wife, Cecily, and their two sons, although he seems just fine with that.

For the latest updates and news on cravings, tips for managing specific cravings, and to stay connected with the Craving community, visit www.facebook.com/CravingBook and follow @CravingBook on Twitter. Hazelden also offers an online social community for those in recovery and their families, at www.hazelden.org/social.

· · ·